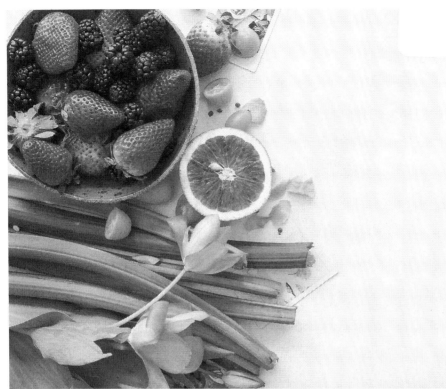
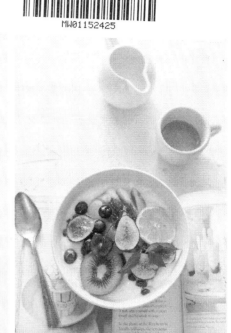
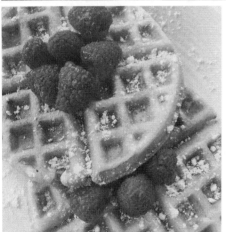
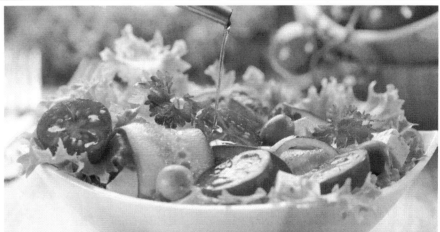

KETO DIET FOR WOMEN AFTER 50

HOW TO HEALTHY LOSE WEIGHT FAST WITH 5 SECRETS TO BURN FAT. INCLUDING TASTY AND YUMMY RECIPES TO RESET YOUR BODY, BOOST YOUR ENERGY AND FEEL YOUNG

KETY WOMACK

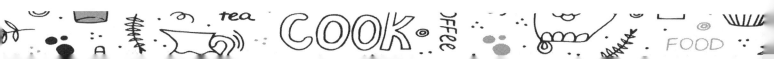

TABLE OF CONTENTS

INTRODUCTION	11
1. IT'S NEVER TOO LATE TO TAKE CARE OF YOURSELF	15
2. DEALING WITH FOOD PROBLEMS	19
3. SIMPLE AND EFFECTIVE METHOD	23
4. NO MORE FASTING AND STOMACH CRAMPS FROM HUNGER DURING THE DAY	27
5. WANT TO LOSE WEIGHT LAZY?	31
6. BAD EATING HABITS WILL NOT IMPROVE YOUR HEALTH	37
7. FOODS YOU SHOULD EAT AND FOODS TO AVOID	41
8. MEAL PLAN AND SHOPPING LIST	45
9. BREAKFAST	49
ALMOND FLOUR KETO PANCAKES	50
KETO COCONUT FLOUR EGG MUFFIN	51
BROCCOLI CHEDDAR CHEESE MUFFINS	52
CHICKEN, BACON, AVOCADO CAESAR SALAD	53
COCONUT MACADAMIA BARS	54
MACADAMIA CHOCOLATE FAT BOMB	55
KETO LEMON BREAKFAST FAT BOMBS	56
BAKED CUSTARD-DAIRY-FREE	57
OLD-FASHIONED BAKED CUSTARD–HEAVY CREAM	58
BACON & EGG FAT BOMBS	59
BEST SCRAMBLED EGGS	60
CREAM CHEESE EGGS	61
HAM & EGG CUPS	62
HAM & SPINACH MINI QUICHE	63

SAUSAGE EGG CASSEROLE   64

SCRAMBLED EGGS WITH MAYO   65

BACON & BRIE FRITTATA   66

JALAPENO POPPERS   67

EGGS BENEDICT DEVILED EGGS   68

10. LUNCH   **69**

CREAM CHEESE STUFFED BABY PEPPERS   70

ARTICHOKE DIP   71

TACO MEAT   72

GREEN BEANS WITH BACON   73

BEEF AND BROCCOLI   74

MEATBALLS   75

RAINBOW MASON JAR SALAD   76

FISH CAKES   77

LASAGNA STUFFED PEPPERS   78

KOREAN GROUND BEEF BOWL   79

SALMON SKEWERS WRAPPED WITH PROSCIUTTO   80

BUFFALO DRUMSTICKS AND CHILI AIOLI   81

SLOW COOKED ROASTED PORK AND CREAMY GRAVY   82

BACON-WRAPPED MEATLOAF   83

LAMB CHOPS AND HERB BUTTER   84

CRISPY CUBAN PORK ROAST   85

KETO BARBECUED RIBS   86

SKINNY BANG BANG ZUCCHINI NOODLES   87

KETO CAESAR SALAD   88

KETO BUFFALO CHICKEN EMPANADAS   89

PEPPERONI AND CHEDDAR STROMBOLI   90

TUNA CASSEROLE   91

BRUSSELS SPROUT AND HAMBURGER GRATIN   92

BACON APPETIZERS   93

11. DINNER — 95

ANGRY ALFREDO FROM OLIVE GARDEN — 96

BEEF BARBACOA AT CHIPOTLE-SLOW-COOKED — 97

BEEF & BROCCOLI FROM PF CHANG'S — 98

CHICKEN SALAD FROM CHICKEN SALAD CHICK — 99

CHIPOTLE GRILL GLUTEN-FREE STEAK BOWL — 100

CHIPOTLE GUACAMOLE SAUCE — 101

CHIPOTLE PORK CARNITAS FROM CHIPOTLE — 102

CRAWFISH ETOUFFEE FROM MAGNOLIA BAR AND GRILL — 103

HASH-BROWN CASSEROLE FROM CRACKER BARREL — 104

SOUTHWESTERN EGG ROLLS FROM CHILIES — 105

LAMB SHANKS — 106

ZUPPA TOSCANA — 107

MEXICAN SHREDDED BEEF — 108

BEEF STEW — 109

COCONUT SHRIMP — 110

CAULIFLOWER RICE SOUP WITH CHICKEN — 111

QUICK PUMPKIN SOUP — 112

FRESH AVOCADO SOUP — 113

CREAMY GARLIC CHICKEN — 114

CAULIFLOWER CHEESECAKE — 115

CHINESE PORK BOWL — 116

TURKEY-PEPPER MIX — 117

12. DRINKS — 119

BRACING GINGER SMOOTHIE — 120

MORNING COFFEE WITH CREAM — 121

BERRY BLAST SMOOTHIE — 122

CHOCOLATE PEANUT BUTTER SMOOTHIE — 123

LOW-CARB STRAWBERRY SMOOTHIE — 124

BLUEBERRY SMOOTHIE — 125

CINNAMON RASPBERRY BREAKFAST SMOOTHIE — 126

CREAMY HOT CHOCOLATE												127

13. SIDES												**129**

ALMOND FLOUR CRACKERS												130

GLUTEN-FREE BAGELS												131

ROASTED CABBAGE WITH LEMON												132

KETO PEANUT BUTTER BALLS												133

SPINACH-MOZZARELLA STUFFED BURGERS												134

AVOCADO TUNA MELT BITES												135

CABBAGE PATTIES												136

COOL & SPICY JICAMA SLAW												137

CREAMY GREEN CABBAGE												138

CREAMY SPINACH-RICH BALLET												139

DRIED BEEF & CREAM CHEESE BALL												140

GARLIC & OLIVE OIL SPAGHETTI SQUASH												141

MARINARA ZOODLES												142

MUSHROOM & CAULIFLOWER RISOTTO												143

RED PEPPER ZOODLES												144

STUFFED MUSHROOMS												145

ZUCCHINI NOODLE GRATIN												146

14. MEAT												**147**

KETO RIB EYE STEAK												148

KETO GROUND BEEF AND GREEN BEANS												149

SPICY BEEF MEATBALLS												150

GARLIC & THYME LAMB CHOPS												151

JAMAICAN JERK PORK ROAST												152

KETO MEATBALLS												153

ROASTED LEG OF LAMB												154

FLAVORFUL PULLED PORK												155

ITALIAN LAMB CHOPS												156

QUICK AND EASY MONGOLIAN BEEF												157

BEEF NOODLE SOUP SPICY KOREAN												158

ASIAN-INSPIRED PORK CHOPS 159

CROCKPOT PORK CHOPS 160

HOT TEX-MEX PORK CASSEROLE 161

MAPLE COUNTRY-STYLE PORK RIBS SLOW-COOKED 162

KOFTA KEBAB 163

15. SEAFOODS **165**

KETO BAKED SALMON WITH LEMON AND BUTTER 166

KETOGENIC SPICY OYSTER 167

GARLIC LIME MAHI-MAHI 168

FISH AND LEEK SAUTÉ 169

SMOKED SALMON SALAD 170

KETO BAKED SALMON WITH PESTO 171

ROASTED SALMON WITH PARMESAN DILL CRUST 172

KETO FRIED SALMON WITH BROCCOLI AND CHEESE 173

TANGY SHRIMP 174

SALMON SUSHI ROLLS 175

SHRIMP LETTUCE WRAPS WITH BUFFALO SAUCE 176

SHRIMP SCAMPI WITH GARLIC 177

BAKED TILAPIA 178

16. POULTRY **179**

BROCCOLI CHEDDAR CHICKEN FROM CRACKER BARREL 180

CHICKEN BAKE FROM COSTCO 181

CHICKEN CASSEROLE FROM CRACKER BARREL 182

CHIPOTLE CHICKEN 183

CHICKEN LETTUCE WRAPS FROM PF CHANG'S 184

CHICKEN PICCATA FROM OLIVE GARDEN 185

EASY MALIBU CHICKEN FROM SIZZLER STEAK HOUSE 186

GARLIC ROSEMARY CHICKEN FROM OLIVE GARDEN 187

INSTANT POT CHICKEN FROM GENERAL TSO'S 188

17. VEGETABLES 189

BRUSSELS SPROUTS WITH BACON 190

MIXED VEGETABLE PATTIES-INSTANT POT 191

EASY ROASTED BROCCOLI 192

BOILED ASPARAGUS WITH SLICED LEMON 193

ROASTED CABBAGE WITH BACON 194

LOADED CAULIFLOWER 195

ZUCCHINI CAULIFLOWER FRITTERS 196

EGGLESS SALAD 197

MOUTH-WATERING GUACAMOLE 198

ROASTED GREEN BEANS 199

FRIED TOFU 200

CURRY ROASTED CAULIFLOWER 201

ROASTED BRUSSELS SPROUTS WITH PECANS AND ALMOND BUTTER 202

18. SOUPS 203

BROCCOLI CHEESE SOUP 204

CAULIFLOWER, LEEK, AND BACON SOUP 205

EGG DROP SOUP 206

FRENCH ONION SOUP 207

CAULIFLOWER FAUX-TATTOOS 208

THAI SHRIMP SOUP 209

ITALIAN SAUSAGE SOUP WITH TOMATOES & ZUCCHINI NOODLES 210

SHIRATAKI SOUP 211

CHILLED CUCUMBER SOUP 212

CREAMY MUSHROOM SOUP 213

BROCCOLI SOUP 214

19. SALADS 215

KALE SALAD WITH THE BACON AND BLUE CHEESE 216

GREEK SALAD WITH VINAIGRETTE SALAD DRESSING 217

BACON AVOCADO SALAD 218

SEARED SQUID SALAD WITH RED CHILI DRESSING 219

CAULIFLOWER AND CASHEW NUT SALAD	220
SALMON AND LETTUCE SALAD	221
PRAWNS SALAD WITH MIXED LETTUCE GREENS	222
POACHED EGG SALAD WITH LETTUCE AND OLIVES	223
REFRESHING CUCUMBER SALAD	224
CABBAGE COCONUT SALAD	225
AVOCADO CABBAGE SALAD	226
TURNIP SALAD	227
BRUSSELS SPROUTS SALAD	228
BEEF SALAD WITH VEGETABLES	229
NIÇOISE SALAD	230
SHRIMP, TOMATO, AND AVOCADO SALAD	231
PESTO CHICKEN SALAD	232
FRESH SUMMER SALAD	233
KETO TACO SALAD	234
20. SNACKS	**235**
BUNLESS BURGER–KETO STYLE	236
SALMON PASTA	237
WRAPPED BACON CHEESEBURGER	238
KETO TORTILLA CHIPS	239
CHEESE JALAPENO BREAD	240
KETO SEED CRACKERS	241
KETO COCONUT PORRIDGE	242
DAIRY-FREE PIZZA	243
LOW CARB BANANA WAFFLES	244
AVOCADO YOGURT DIP	245
CHEESE BALLS	246
SPICY CHICKEN THIGHS	247
CORNED BEEF AND CAULIFLOWER HASH	248
LOW CARB GNOCCHI	249
AVOCADO FRIES	250

21. DESSERTS ... **251**

MOCHA MOUSSE ... 252

STRAWBERRY RHUBARB CUSTARD ... 253

CRÈME BRULEE ... 254

PUMPKIN PIE PUDDING ... 255

CHOCOLATE MUFFINS ... 256

LEMON FAT BOMBS ... 257

VANILLA FROZEN YOGURT ... 258

ICE CREAM ... 259

RASPBERRY MOUSSE ... 260

CHOCOLATE SPREAD WITH HAZELNUTS ... 261

QUICK AND SIMPLE BROWNIE ... 262

CUTE PEANUT BALLS ... 263

TURKEY CARROT MUSHROOM DUMPLINGS ... 264

LEMON BREAD FROM STARBUCKS ... 265

MOLTEN CHOCOLATE CAKE FROM CHILI'S ... 266

CONCLUSION ... **267**

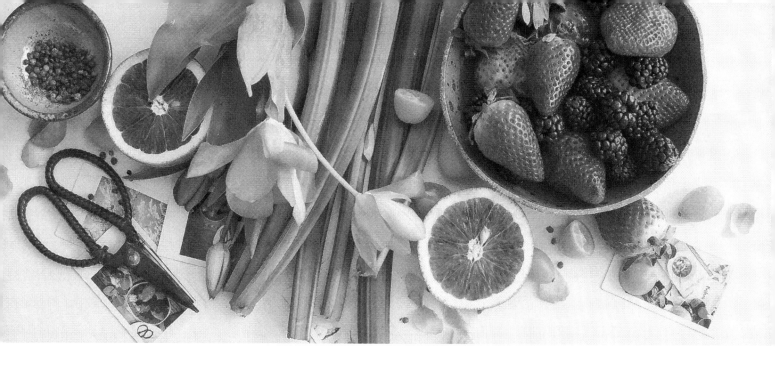

INTRODUCTION

Keto diet is a low-carb diet plan in which you eat a very low amount of carbs and a high amount of fat on a weekly basis. The term itself is derived from the Ketogenic state which is a condition due to ketones build up in the body to supply the necessary energy as glycogen stores become depleted.

Ketosis is the metabolic state in which your body uses fat instead of protein for energy. Your body becomes a fat-burning machine since fat is the only form of energy your body can use. Most of the fuel that your body uses for energy is derived from carbohydrates. The carb intake has to be controlled as you want to jump to a state of Ketosis and avoid health issues. This is one of the most controversial diets and has become an obsession for some people.

Ketogenic Technique Levels

The standard Ketogenic diet (SKD) comprises moderate proteins with high-fat content and maintains low carbs. The averages vary, but the ratio usually operates using 5% on carbs, 75% for high-fat, and 20% for your protein counts.

The targeted keto diet, which is also called TKD, will provide you with a technique to add carbs to the diet plan while working out or are more active.

The cyclical Ketogenic diet (CKD) entails a restricted five-day keto diet plan followed by two high-carbohydrate days.

The high-protein keto diet is comparable to the standard keto plan (SKD) in all aspects, except you will consume more protein.

Scientific Ketogenic Benefits

- Accelerated Fat Loss for Overweight & Obese Individuals: Weight Loss and Anti-Aging is improved long term according to a Harvard Study in 2018. Those who participate in the keto's intermittent fasting phase diet plan may exceed healthy figures when it comes to weight. It is imperative to use the keto diet plan to get started on the right path for weight loss.

- Epileptic Seizures: For children, reductions in seizures have occurred for children who have used the keto diet. The therapeutic keto diet used for epilepsy often restricts the carbs to fewer than 15grams of carbs daily to further escalate your ketone levels. Don't try to reach these levels unless you have the supervision of a medical professional.

- Dravet Syndrome, a severe form of epilepsy, is marked by prolonged, uncontrollable, and frequent seizures. Currently, available medications don't improve symptoms in about 1/3 of the Dravet Syndrome patients. A clinical study used 13 children with the syndrome to stay on the Ketogenic diet for more than one year to remain seizure-free. Over 50% of the group decreased in the frequency of the seizures. It was reported that six of the patients stopped the diet later, and one remains seizure-free.

- Improvement of Your Cholesterol Profile: An arterial buildup is typically associated with triglyceride and cholesterol levels, proven to improve with the keto diet plan. Cut down your chance of heart disease. The triglycerides found in large amounts in carbohydrates are also found in high concentrations in those who have experienced cardiovascular problems.

- Blood Pressure Levels Lowered: When you begin the Ketogenic diet, your blood pressure may become lower, making you feel dizzy at first. Don't worry or feel overly concerned because that's a clear indication that the carbohydrates are working. However, suppose you are currently taking medications. It's a good idea to speak with your physician about the possibility of lowering some of your doses during the time that you are on the Ketogenic plan.

- Regulate Your Blood Sugar: According to a London 2005 Study, the Ketogenic diet can help reduce the "bad" LDL cholesterol, inflammatory markers, blood triglycerides, and blood sugar for those with type 2 diabetes.

- Polycystic Ovary Syndrome (PCOS) Improves: This is an endocrine disorder affecting young women of childbearing years. It is also associated with insulin resistance, obesity, and hyperinsulinemia. A 6-month study concluded a significant improvement in weight loss in fasting women over 24 weeks. The group limited carb intake to 20grams daily for 24 weeks.

The Ketogenic plan also helps other conditions, including Alzheimer' Disease, Parkinson's Disease, chronic inflammation, and migraines.

Ketogenic 'Good' Fats

You have many options to receive fats that will not have a 'bad' effect on your Ketogenic diet. Select organic oil, including red palm oil, avocado, sesame, olive, and flaxseed oil. Also, select other fats, including unsalted butter, chicken fat, duck fat, and beef tallow.

Olive oil dates back for centuries to a time where oil was used for anointing kings and priests. It's a high-quality oil maintaining low-acidity, making this oil have a smoke point as high as 410° Fahrenheit. That's higher than most cooking applications call for, making olive oil more heat-stable than many other cooking fats. It contains zero carbs for two teaspoons.

Monounsaturated fats, such as olive oil, are also linked with better blood sugar regulation, including lower fasting glucose and reducing inflammation throughout the body. Olive oil also helps to prevent cardiovascular disease. It protects your vascular system's integrity by lowering LDL, which is also called your 'bad' cholesterol. You can choose olives at one net carb for three jumbo—5 large/10 small.

Purchase macadamia oil for its high smoke point of 390° Fahrenheit. It carries a mild flavor, which is a super alternative for olive oil in mayonnaise.

Ghee has zero carbs for one teaspoon. Unsweetened flaked coconut is only two net carbs for 3 tbsp.

1. IT'S NEVER TOO LATE TO TAKE CARE OF YOURSELF

You've decided this is the right time in your life to get serious about weight loss and wellness. You've chosen the Ketogenic diet as the vehicle you'll use to reach your goals. You have unique reasons, objectives you will be working toward, and benefits you are already looking forward to enjoying.

To set the stage for getting started, take some time to reflect on your ground zero or starting point. Make some notes about why you feel ready now and what caused you to choose keto here at the beginning of this journey.

Make a note of your goals. It's okay to set a long-term objective to work toward achieving. But research indicates when you set specific, short-term, reasonable goals along the way, you'll have a greater likelihood of reaching them.

If you have any pounds to drop, you can think about the total you want to shed or the goal weight you'd like to end up reaching. But if you're only looking at the long-term goal, it could feel a little bit overwhelming to you.

Specific goals are laser-focused on a singular thing. A particular objective might be to lose five pounds or keep your carb intake to 20grams per day or less. Those are much more likely to keep you fully engaged than broad or general goals like, "I want to lose weight" or "My goal is to limit my carbohydrates." Keeping your goals focused on a specific thing will lead to more effective planning and tracking toward your goal.

Measurable goals make it easy to evaluate your success. For example, looking at the two examples above, the broad goal of "I want to lose weight" is hard to measure because it's not specific enough. Will you be happy if you lose one pound, or will you be disappointed with a one-pound loss? Adding the quantifier and making the goal specific, "My goal is to lose five pounds, "you'll be able to measure when you've successfully reached that goal easily. In the example, "I want to limit my carbohydrates,' 'limit' can mean many things, making it hard to evaluate progress. Using the more specific version, "I want to limit my daily carbohydrate intake to 20grams or less," will remove the ambiguity and allow you to hone in on that exact desired outcome.

Achievable goals are realistic and practical. Let's say you have a wedding or special event coming up in eight weeks. You could set a goal of losing forty pounds, an average of five pounds per week for eight weeks. The problem is, having a plan to drop weight at a rapid rate could set you up disappointed if you don't reach that milestone. Why not choose something that feels doable, like losing four pounds per month? You are much more apt to stay the course if you think you can realistically manage what it will take to realize that goal. Feeling confident that you can reasonably accomplish what you have set as a goal is a big motivator and increases your success.

Relevant goals should get you one step closer to your desired outcome and align with your long-term goals. They should also align with your values. If you value overall wellness and nutrition, your action steps will align with that and nudge you to eat well. If your long-term goal is to get within your recommended weight ranges for your age, weight, height, and gender, your short-term goals along the way should support that desired result.

Time-based goals have an estimated achievement date. It's one thing to say, "I want to lose five pounds." But when you put an achievement date on that goal, the goal changes. You might say, "I want to lose five pounds within my first two weeks on keto. You can easily track your progress for that goal, which motivates you to stay engaged. This short-term goal, too, should be reasonable and achievable. Setting your desired achievement date too far out could serve as demotivation instead of inspiration. "My goal is to shed five pounds in one year" is not going to challenge you to work hard for your goal. Conversely, having a plan to lose five pounds in two days might be too aggressive and set you up to fail or feel discouraged.

If you'll take time to consider both your long-term and short-term goals thoughtfully, and if you are intentional about making them specific, measurable, attainable, relevant, and time-bound, you'll be setting yourself up to win!

Physical and Mental Benefits

How keto helps you eat well every day, lose weight at a good pace, and supports your overall good health.

You've already seen this sentence several times in this book. That's because it represents our hope for you. That the tools in these pages will equip and empower you to do just that—to eat well every day, lose weight at a good pace, and enjoy overall good health. Let's dive in and break down all three pieces of this puzzle.

Eat Well Every Day

You might have arrived here in this place because your eating habits haven't been the best. Perhaps you have a sweet tooth and consume more sugar than is healthy. Maybe you struggle with breaking old dieting habits, like avoiding fats but loading up on carbs. Or it could be that you've just never applied yourself to a healthy pattern of eating.

No matter where you're starting, you can begin to eat well every day, and after you've been eating well every day for a few weeks, you'll be astounded at the positive changes in how you look, feel, think and perform.

When you eat well every day, your sleep will feel more restful, your hair, nails, and skin will both look and feel better, and you'll notice your body functioning at its best. You'll enjoy increased mental sharpness, improved mood, higher energy levels. You'll begin to see some improvements to specific health conditions. For those with diabetes, you might notice your blood sugar readings and A1C results are better. For those with hypertension, you might see more manageable blood pressure readings.

Eating well every day helps you look better, feel better, and function better in your body's complex supportive systems. The keto plan nudges you toward this healthy pattern by recommending the foods that best support your health, and away from those junk food, highly processed, or super sweet foods that are carb-rich and nutrient-poor.

Lose Weight at a Good Pace

One of the first questions dieters ask is, "How much weight will I lose per week?" This question is impossible to resolve because each individual has a wide variety of factors that can influence the rate of weight loss. Your metabolism isn't exactly like everyone else's. You might have preexisting medical considerations that impact your weight loss pace. If you have a substantial number of pounds lot to lose, you might notice a pretty rapid weight loss pattern, especially at the beginning of your journey. If you have a more modest number of pounds to lose to be within normal weight ranges, your rate might be slower.

Most diets suggest that if you follow the plan faithfully and follow a regular exercise regime, you could expect to lose anywhere from half a pound to two pounds per week.

It's not uncommon for dieters to experience a weight loss of two to ten pounds in the first week to ten days. That's because, in the early days, when you begin limiting your carb intake, your body releases a lot of water. This water weight loss is not the fat loss you'll experience later on, but it's a loss on the scale just the same, and a significant one.

This initial loss happens because carbohydrates need a water supply to stay in your body. Your body doesn't immediately use glucose for energy. Instead, it stores it in your muscles in the form of glycogen. Glycogen binds to water, so when you first start limiting your carbs, your body will use up that glycogen reserve first before it starts burning fat instead. Once it has exhausted its supply of glycogen, the water reserved for storage gets eliminated. So, the number on your scale can move in a big way during the first week or two on keto.

This rapid loss at the beginning is evidence of a strong start and means you are well on your way to being in ketosis. You need to be attentive to hydration, though, as your rapid water loss could lead to dehydration or constipation. Plan to increase your water intake to keep things moving and make sure you don't dehydrate.

Most experts report a save average rate of loss is between one and two pounds per week. Most keto followers lose the fattest in the first two to three months of the keto diet, although your weight/fat loss can continue as long as you consistently follow the diet. You already know that your pace varies based on how long you follow the plan, how much weight you hope to lose, and your overall health condition. Be encouraged that at the end of a month, six months, or a year, you will enjoy significant improvements to your overall health by losing weight and eating well every day.

Enjoy Better Health in General

Losing excess weight helps you look and feel better, which is precisely what most people are looking for when they begin to follow the keto diet plan. The benefits are worth it!

Following keto can help you have healthier hair, skin, and nails. You will enjoy more mental clarity and more energy. You'll feel satisfied and experience fewer cravings on keto, and eating well every day will lower the inflammation present in your body and reduce your risks for chronic diseases.

While the feedback you get from the scale is certainly one way to measure your success, it's not the only way. You're likely to notice the changes in the mirror just as you see the changes on the scale. You can expect to both feel better and look better in your clothes, sure, but you can also look forward to receiving a favorable report from your doctor as your blood lipid profile changes.

The keto diet fills your toolbox with everything you need to achieve an overall healthier lifestyle.

Is Healthier Eating Happier Eating?

Did you know there is an increasing body of evidence proving the connection between healthy habits around eating and overall happiness? You might have the notion that eating pizza, birthday cake, ice cream, and potato chips makes you happy. For many, those are the kinds of comfort foods that are go-to choices when a little pick-me-up is needed. But the contrary is true. Consuming unhealthy comfort foods can trigger a negative chain of events.

Often, consuming highly processed foods, especially those packed with added sugar, can cause you to seem sluggish, lazy, and sick afterward. In addition to those physical reactions, you might experience emotional responses too. You might feel disappointed in yourself for overindulging in something you knew wasn't an excellent choice for your body. You might feel defeated or like you failed and discouraged that you might never get this under control. You might be sad because of how unhealthy you feel after a junk food binge.

The opposite is true, as well. Research confirms that making healthy food choices can contribute to your overall feelings of happiness. Research also confirms that happier people make healthier choices.

So, imagine the impact on your success if you can bring those negative chains of events to a screeching halt and begin to enjoy that chain of events that gives you happy feelings when you make healthy food choices. You will feel incentivized to make healthy food choices again. There is no way to overstate the crucial role that eating healthy every day plays in your overall quality of life.

2. DEALING WITH FOOD PROBLEMS

Trying to lose weight can be intimidating at any age. However, once you're in your fifties, it becomes even more overwhelming. Most of us know this happens, but only a few know why. After 25, which is when the body stops bone growth, the metabolic rate goes down by about 2% every ten years. So, the amount of calories you can consume without gaining weight also decreases with each decade. This is why it is important to increase your levels of activity and be more conscious of your food intake.

As you grow older, it becomes more difficult to lose weight as easily as, say, five years before, and because of this, most people lose hope of dropping weight as they grow.

Here are a few ways you can start your keto diet:

Set a Date

Planning a date to start your Keto journey doesn't necessarily mean you need a date to go shopping or meal prepping. It means that you will prepare yourself mentally for the change in your lifestyle. This also means letting your loved ones know that you will soon embark on this journey that may or may not be easy and that you will need their support and encouragement. Informing people around you about your lifestyle change encourages them to be more thoughtful and considerate about your dietary restrictions, and they might create dinner or lunch plans with you according to your new lifestyle.

Create a Routine

Adopting a good routine, especially in the morning, can help you on your journey. Start your day by drinking plenty of water and consuming a teaspoon of coconut oil. Make sure that you get a good night's sleep and stay active during the day, as well as taking some time out daily to exercise.

Get Rid of Non-Keto Foods

Most of us are guilty of indulging in unhealthy foods a few days before we embark on this Ketogenic weight loss journey. To avoid this from happening, throw away all non-Ketogenic foods from your food cabinets and refrigerator. A mistake that most of us make when starting a healthier diet is to think that the motivation of losing weight will be the same throughout, and you won't be tempted to eat that chocolate bar lying around in your refrigerator. However, adopting a healthy lifestyle and being consistent can challenge, so to not risk indulging in guilty pleasures, it is best to get rid of all non-keto foods from your life and home.

Try Intermittent Fasting

Intermittent fasting is considered being a foolproof way to control your intake of carbohydrates effectively. Intermittent fasting may seem scary to most people, as we talk about a certain number of hours without consuming foods. A great way to go about it without letting it seem too daunting, and instead of counting hours, you just have to skip one meal every day. Most doctors suggest having a late breakfast or brunch and an early dinner later on. This automatically creates a fast of 12 to 13 hours.

Consume Less Than 25grams of Carbs Daily

To get your body to transition to ketosis and be motivated into burning fat, you need to increase your intake of healthy fats and lower your intake of carbohydrates. It is recommended to keep your carbohydrate consumption to less than 25grams a day. Start leaning towards healthy fats and proteins, such as coconut oil, avocados, and eggs. When the body gets more fats and fewer carbs, it has a good balance, and there isn't a lack of ketones.

Counting Carbs for Beginners

Perhaps the most impressive aspect of keto is learning how to control your carbs. But here's the thing, you may have some limitations when you're only a beginner. In the beginning, stick to a total of 20grams of net carbs each day. We have explained how to calculate net carbs in the later chapters (net carbs are absorbed). This milestone is usually the starting point for most people as they start keto for the first time.

We urge you to stick to these guidelines and follow them for at least three months. For the keto diet to work, you'll need to make sure your body's going through ketosis. One of the most reliable ways to test this is by regularly checking your blood with a blood ketone testing meter. (If you're planning on switching to keto for the long run, this is an investment worth making).

Your blood ketone levels should rise to 0.1 mmol/L when you're new to the diet. 0.5 mmol/L is the stage that indicates that you're in ketosis now.

The good old keto flu is another sign that indicates the diet is working (we'll talk about the keto flu in detail in the later chapters).

What Is Your Carbs Limit?

This is the minimal amount of carbs you can consume without kicking out your body from the state of ketosis.

Factors That May Affect Your Daily Carb Limit

Now here's the thing, your daily carb limit isn't set to stone and can be influenced by many factors. Here are some factors which you might need to take into account:

Emotional Stress

Emotional stress can alter insulin response and a whole bunch of stress hormones. So, your blood glucose level might be particularly high on a stressful day. This will get in the way of the ketone on your body. To maintain a healthy lifestyle, practice ways to manage stress, you can go for a long walk or talk to a friend. Learning how to manage stress is an excellent way to take care of your overall well-being.

Exercising and Heavy Workouts

Exercise, particularly long and tedious workouts, can influence your glucose levels in many ways. Performing intense workouts without taking breaks can raise cortisol levels that also impact glucose and increase blood levels. This is why it is important to rest and allow your body enough time to recover.

Also, you might experience a sudden spike in glucose levels after working out. This is normal and will tend to subside after an hour or so. That being said, seniors are better off practicing lightweight exercises that will burn more fats and help them reach ketosis much faster.

Coffee can also affect insulin levels in the body. For instance, some people might experience a spike in glucose levels, while others may find that coffee helps with insulin sensitivity. If you're a fan of caffeine, we suggest you test your glucose levels 30 minutes before having a cup and 30 minutes after.

Sleep Cycle

Research conducted by Cedars-Sinai Medical Center in Los Angeles, CA, has indicated how sleep deprivation is known to hamper fasting insulin sensitivity. So, if you're not getting enough sleep, you might experience a change in your blood glucose levels. If you're interested in testing this hypothesis, simply check your blood glucose levels with a full night's sleep and once when your sleep's been interrupted.

Understanding How to Calculate Net Carbs

If you're new to the whole keto frenzy, you're probably wondering how you should calculate your carbs. Before we get a touch down on the specifics, it's important to understand what net carbs are. This is a term that you are likely to come across when looking at food nutrition labels. When browsing true nutrition labels, you will find sugar, alcohol, and fiber under the carbohydrate category.

What Are Net Carbs?

To find out your daily carb count, you will need to keep track of the net carbs that you are consuming. The term 'net carbs' refers to carbohydrates absorbed by the body and utilized for energy. It's important to understand that not all carbohydrates, such as insoluble fiber, spike up blood sugar levels; hence you don't have to keep track of these substances when counting carbs.

How to Calculate Net Carbs?

One simple way to calculate the number of net carbs in whole foods is to subtract the fiber content from the total number of carbohydrates. When calculating net carbs for processed foods, you'll have to subtract the number of fiber and sugar alcohols from total carbs.

- Fiber: Though fiber is a type of carbohydrate found in plants, your body doesn't have the enzyme to digest it. Hence, the fiber content you consume is digested without any change. Subtract out the fiber content from the total carbohydrates count, and you're good to go.

- Sugar alcohols: While sugar alcohols such as erythritol and xylitol taste sweet, they are only partially digested by the body and largely remain indigestible. Hence when buying food, you can quickly subtract the sugar alcohol content from the total number of carbohydrates.

However, it's important to note that not all sugar alcohols are completely carb-free. Here's where you'll need to be wary of manufacturers who forcefully try to make their products seem lower carb than they are.

You can easily combat this problem by being aware of the different types of sugar alcohol. Xylitol, erythritol, lactitol and mannitol are sugar alcohols that you don't have to count when calculating net carbs.

Maltitol, isomalt, glycerin and sorbitol count as about half a gram carb. When counting these sugar alcohols, all you have to do is take the total number of grams and divide it by 2.

A simple way to depict this equation is through:

Net carbs = total carbs–fiber–sugar alcohols + (maltitol, isomalt, glycerin and sorbitol/ 2)

It is important to calculate these carbs, as Keto requires you to count every single gram of carbohydrate you consume.

3. SIMPLE AND EFFECTIVE METHOD

The Ketogenic diet provides the body with premium fuel in facts that make you fitter and younger with the energy of a twenty-year-old and the best part, it lasts longer than carb fuel.

By following the Ketogenic diet, you can lose all the unwanted weight without ever stepping foot in a gym, with no meal portion control or counting calories. The Ketogenic diet has proven to work for people with many backgrounds and health issues like having blood sugar issues, obesity, post-pregnancy, food addictions, suffering from emotional eating, etc. Before going into more details about the keto diet, specifically for seniors over 50, let's dive into its history.

The Ketogenic diet is nothing new; it has existed for over ninety years. Dr. Russell Wilder designed the Keto diet in 1924 as a treatment for epileptic patients. He found out that fasting, which led the body into ketosis, proved fruitful to control the epileptic seizures in their patient, but fasting wasn't a permanent solution. Hence, they came up with a high-fat and low-carb diet for the patients that worked equally and that too effectively as a cure for epilepsy when no medicine could help. With more research on this diet, the keto diet began being successfully used to treat various other medical conditions, especially obesity. Other benefits apart from epilepsy and losing a few pounds of weights are:

- Alzheimer's disease

- Parkinson's disease

- Multiple Sclerosis

- Healing traumatic brain injuries

- Improve cardiovascular health

- Prevent heart attack and stroke

- Reduce and maintain healthy blood sugar levels

- Fight various kinds of cancer

- Treat Autism

- Decrease acne

- Decrease risk factors for polycystic ovary syndrome and respiratory disease

Our body functions and performs its processes differently at an old age compared to when it is 20 or 30 years old because, at this age, the metabolism is too slow to burn off any extra calories or fats. Unfortunately, this is a sad reality, but it doesn't mean that a person over 50 cannot implement a Ketogenic lifestyle. Of course, the Ketogenic diet is varied, and you have to make a few changes in it and adjust to it precisely.

A Ketogenic diet supports very low or zero-carbs in the diet. And this is not good in the initial days when the body is transitioning to a Keto diet. We have always been eating so many carbs that handling this sudden change in our body's food gets challenging, and you end up suffering from Keto flu. And with more age, your body has a harder time adjusting and overcoming the side effects of adapting to the keto diet. The younger generation has a robust support system, but over 50, the side effect hits you harder, and you take more time to recover. You may experience fatigue, headache, nausea, dizziness, lack of motivation and difficulty in focusing. These symptoms are enough to discourage anyone who is finally ready to take charge of their health and body once again, and this stops you from getting the healthy changes you deserve. But don't feel low and worried. Even at this age, the keto diet will work fine for you, and you can still use all the incredible benefits of the Ketogenic diet.

Do you know that eating more fats during a Ketogenic diet might prevent you from having a heart stroke?? Why? There is a general misconception that fats clog arteries, but that is not the Ketogenic diet because you burn fats on the keto diet and lose weight.

5 Simple Rules

Here are some simple rules that always work for adhering to the Ketogenic diet with no difficulty and headache.

Rule #1: No Carbs

The primary aim of the Ketogenic diet is to have carbs as low as possible. You cannot consume foods that are high in carbs, except for veggies. In the initial days of your Ketogenic diet, you can stick to 5 to 10 percent of carbs in your meals, about 20grams, not more than that or else your body will take a lot of time to get into ketosis. And with time, decrease the carbs and go to zero levels.

Rule #2: Have a Fatty Meal

Most of the keto-ers fail to realize that they should load their body with as many fats as possible during the first meal of the day —breakfast. For example, you can have a quick fatty breakfast in keto coffee mixed with MCT oil or high-fat butter. Or, you can have your regular breakfast consisting of eggs, bacon, and avocado. Your goal should be to get one-third portion of fat for the day from breakfast. For the rest of the day, get most of the fat from fatty meats, cheeses, nuts, avocado oil, one or two cups of salad greens and coconut milk.

Rule #3: Don't Go High in Protein

The Ketogenic diet allows just enough protein essential to maintain growth; it's not a high-protein diet. You will take the time to know the right amount of protein you should consume in the beginning. However, you can start with having grass-fed and fatty meat about a fist, twice a day. This rule of getting protein into your body is not perfect, but it is a simple starting point until you figure out how much protein you need. The best fatty meats are beef, skin-on chicken thighs, pork, salmon, lamb, wild games and eggs. Remember that you cannot have too much meat on the keto diet. Start with taking two fists amount of meat regularly and then cut back to one and a half fist.

Rule #4: Don't Restrict Calories

The significant benefit of the keto diet is its inadvertent calorie restriction. If you are not convinced of this, then try this rule for three weeks. For three weeks, don't do a calorie count of your meals and don't weigh and measure. Eat until you are satisfied and not hungry anymore; don't eat until you are bursting. After three weeks, check your weight, and if it declines, then keep following this rule.

Rule #5: Track and Adjust

If you follow the above four rules to the T, your body should get into ketosis and start losing fat. To make sure you are doing it right and successfully, you need to do some tracking of whatever you are doing to achieve your goal. The easiest way is to track your weight, which means if you are losing weight, you are doing it right. The next easiest way is through the smell of your breath by using a breath analyzer. You can also check ketones level with ketone pee strips. Ketones are excreted out of the body through urine, and the ketone strips change their color based on the level of ketosis your body is in. Another way is to get a blood ketone test that will show whether your body is in ketosis, and in this way, you will know how successful you are sticking to the keto diet.

Follow these five rules and have no problem getting your body into ketosis and staying in this state. The three to four weeks might be a little rough, but if you are stuck with keto as closely as possible, you will find that the keto diet is easy to live on and its amazing wonders. Once you are there and the fat-burning is built, you are good to go.

4. NO MORE FASTING AND STOMACH CRAMPS FROM HUNGER DURING THE DAY

Losing Weight

For most people, this is the foremost benefit of switching to keto! Their previous diet method may have stalled for them, or they were noticing weight creeping back on. With keto, studies have shown that people have been able to follow this diet and relay fewer hunger pangs and suppressed appetite while losing weight at the same time! You are minimizing your carbohydrate intake, which means fewer blood sugar spikes. Often, those fluctuations in blood sugar levels make you feel hungrier and more prone to snacking in between meals. Instead, by guiding the body towards ketosis, you are eating a more fulfilling diet of fat and protein and harnessing energy from ketone molecules instead of glucose. Studies show that low-carb diets effectively reduce visceral fat (the fat you commonly see around the abdomen increases as you become obese). This reduces your risk of obesity and improves your health in the long-term.

Reduce the Risk of Type 2 Diabetes

The problem with carbohydrates is how unstable they make blood sugar levels. This can be very dangerous for people who have diabetes or are pre-diabetic because of unstable blood sugar levels or family history. Keto is a great option because of the minimal intake of carbohydrates it requires. Instead, you are harnessing most of your calories from fat or protein, which will not cause blood sugar spikes and, ultimately, pressure the pancreas to secrete insulin. Many studies have found that diabetes patients who followed the keto diet lost more weight and ultimately reduced their fasting glucose levels. This is monumental news for patients who have unstable blood sugar levels or hope to avoid or reduce their diabetes medication intake.

Improve Cardiovascular Risk Symptoms to Overall Lower Your Chances of Having Heart Disease

Most people assume that following a keto diet that is so high in fat content has to increase your risk of coronary heart disease or heart attack, but the research proves otherwise! Research shows that switching to keto can lower your blood pressure, increase your HDL good cholesterol, and reduce your triglyceride fatty acid levels. That's because the fats you are consuming on keto are healthy and high-quality fats, so they reverse many unhealthy symptoms of heart disease. They boost your "good" HDL cholesterol levels and decrease your "bad" LDL cholesterol levels. It also decreases the level of triglyceride fatty acids in the bloodstream. A high level of these can lead to stroke, heart attack, or premature death. And what are the high levels of fatty acids linked to?

Low Consumption of Carbohydrates

With the keto diet, you are drastically cutting your carbohydrate intake to improve fatty acid levels and improve other risk factors. A 2018 study on the keto diet found that it can improve 22 out of 26 risk factors for cardiovascular heart disease! These factors can be very important to some people, especially those who have a history of heart disease in their family.

Increases the Body's Energy Levels

Let's briefly compare the difference between the glucose molecules synthesized from a high carbohydrate intake versus ketones produced on the keto diet. The liver makes ketones and use fat molecules you already stored. This makes them much more energy-rich and a lasting fuel source than glucose, a simple sugar molecule. These ketones can physically and mentally give you a burst of energy, allowing you to have greater focus, clarity, and attention to detail.

Decreases Inflammation in the Body

Inflammation on its own is a natural response by the body's immune system, but when it becomes uncontrollable, it can lead to an array of health problems, some severe and some minor. The health concerns include acne, autoimmune conditions, arthritis, psoriasis, irritable bowel syndrome, and even acne and eczema. Often removing sugars and carbohydrates from your diet can help patients of these diseases avoid flare-ups—and the delightful news is keto does just that! A 2008 research study found that keto decreased a blood marker linked to high inflammation in the body by nearly 40%. This is glorious news for people who may suffer from inflammatory disease and want to change their diet to see improvement.

Increases Your Mental Functioning Level

As we mentioned earlier, the energy-rich ketones can boost the body's physical and mental alertness levels. Research has shown that keto is a much better energy source for the brain than simple sugar glucose molecules are. With nearly 75% of your diet coming from healthy fats, the brain's neural cells and mitochondria have a better energy source to function at the highest level. Some studies have tested patients on the keto diet and found they had higher cognitive functioning, better memory recall, and less memory loss. The keto diet can even decrease the occurrence of migraines, which can be very detrimental to patients.

The Calorie and Nutrient Balance

Do you know why else the Ketogenic Diet is good for you, specifically, as someone who just hit 50 years old? You should keep in mind that as a person advances in age, their calorie needs to decrease. For example, instead of 2,000 calories per day, you'll need only 1,800 calories per day. Why is that? Well, when we start to get old, our physical activity significantly decreases. Hence, we don't need as much energy in our system. However, that doesn't mean our nutrient needs also go down. We still need the same amount of vitamins and minerals.

The Ketogenic Diet manages to hit a balance between these two needs. You get high nutrition for every calorie you get—which means that you'll maintain a decent amount of weight without feeling less energetic for day to day activities.

Heart Diseases

Keto diets help women over 50 to shed those extra pounds. Reducing any amount of weight greatly reduces the chances of a heart attack or any other heart complications. Through the carefully selected diet routine, you are not only losing weight and enjoying delicious meals, but you are significantly boosting your heart's health and reviving yourself from the otherwise dull state that you may have been in before.

Diabetes Control

The careful selection of ingredients, when cooked together, provide rich nutrients, free from any processed or harmful contents such as sugar. Add to that the fact that keto automatically controls your insulin levels. The result is a glucose level that is always under control, and continued control would lead to a day where you will say goodbye to the medications you might be taking for diabetes.

5. WANT TO LOSE WEIGHT LAZY?

If you belong to the population of women over the age of 50, you may be much more involved in weight loss than you were at 30.

There are several diet choices available to help lose weight, but the Ketogenic diet has been among the most common lately. To make the body burn its fat resources more effectively, Keto is a diet that involves reducing carbohydrates and growing fats. Analysis has shown that keto diets are good for general health and weight reduction. Keto diets have facilitated certain individuals to lose excess body fat without extreme desires characteristic of most diets. Any patients with type 2 diabetes have already been shown to use Keto to manage their symptoms. The core of the keto diet is ketones.

As an alternative energy source, the body creates ketones, a fuel compound, while the body is low on blood sugar. Ketones are created when you lower the carb consumption and eat just the correct amount of protein. The Human liver will convert body fat into ketones as you consume keto-friendly foods, which are then used by your body as an energy supply. You are in ketosis as the body uses fat for energy supply. In certain situations, this causes the body to raise its fat-burning, eliminating pockets of unnecessary fat significantly. This fat-burning approach not only lets you shed weight, but it can also fend off cravings during the day and eliminate sugar crashes.

How to Improve the Shape of Your Body with the Right Foods

While it is convenient to tell that the keto diet is higher in fat and lower in carbohydrates, it still feels a little more difficult when you are in the supermarket aisle.

Typically, a Ketogenic diet reduces carbs to 20-50grams a day. Although this can sound daunting, many healthy items will comfortably blend into this form of eating. Safe things to consume on a Ketogenic diet are mentioned below.

Seafood

Fish and shellfish are keto-friendly things. Salmon and other fish are abundant and nearly carb-free in B vitamins, potassium, and selenium. Many seafood forms are carb-free or very poor in carbohydrates. Some healthy sources of vitamins, nutrients, and omega-3s include seafood and shellfish.

Low-Carb Vegetables

Non-starchy foods, like vitamin C and other minerals, are poor in calories and carbohydrates yet rich in several nutrients. For higher-carb diets, low-carb vegetables make perfect replacements. Cauliflower, for example, can imitate rice or mashed potatoes, zucchini can make 'Zoodles,' and spaghetti squash is a suitable replacement for spaghetti.

Cheese

The cheese is healthy and tasty. Hundreds of varieties of cheese are available. Luckily, they are all really low in carbohydrates and strong in fat, making them a perfect choice for a Ketogenic diet. 1gram of carbohydrates, 7grams of protein, and 20 percent of the RDI for calcium is given by one ounce (28grams) of cheddar cheese (20).

Avocados

Avocados are amazingly safe. Avocados are rich in fiber and several nutrients, including potassium, and produce 2grams of net carbs per serving. They can enhance markers of cardiac health.

Meat and Poultry

Meat and poultry on a Ketogenic diet are called staple items. There are no calories in fresh meat and poultry, and they are high in B vitamins and some minerals, including potassium, selenium, and zinc. There are no sugars in meat and poultry, and they are abundant in high-quality protein and a variety of nutrients. The healthiest range is grass-fed beef.

Eggs

Eggs are one of the planet's healthiest and most flexible crops. Eggs each have less than 1gram of carbohydrate and will help you remain full for hours. They are also rich in different nutrients and may help protect the protection of the eyes and core.

Coconut Oil

There are distinctive properties of coconut oil that render it well adapted to a Ketogenic diet. Coconut oil is abundant in MCTs, which can increase the output of ketones. In comparison, metabolic rates can be improved, and weight reduction and abdominal fat can be encouraged.

Plain Greek Yogurt and Cottage Cheese

Per cup, both plain Greek yogurt and cottage cheese produce 5grams of carbs. Analysis has shown that they tend to suppress hunger and facilitate fullness.

Olive Oil

Olive oil supplies the core with impressive benefits. High in heart-healthy monounsaturated fats and antioxidants, extra-virgin olive oil is high. It's great for incorporating salad dressings, mayonnaise, and fried meats.

Nuts and Seeds

Balanced, high-fat, and low-carb foods contain nuts and seeds.

A decreased incidence of coronary failure, some tumors, depression, and other chronic diseases has been correlated with daily nut intake. Nuts and seeds are rich in antioxidants, heart-healthy, and can contribute to healthier aging. They have 0-8grams per ounce of net carbohydrates.

Berries

Many fruits are too rich in carbohydrates to be included in a Ketogenic diet, but an exception is berries.

Berries are low in carbohydrates and strong in fiber content. Berries are nutrient-rich, which can decrease the likelihood of disease. Per the 3.5-ounce portion, they have 5-12grams of net carbs.

Butter and Cream

Butter and cream are great fats that can be used in a Ketogenic diet. Each includes just trace quantities per serving of carbohydrates. Butter and cream are almost carb-free and tend, when eaten in moderation, to have a supportive or positive impact on cardiac health.

Shirataki Noodles

A wonderful contribution to a Ketogenic diet is Shirataki noodles. Noodles from Shirataki produce less than 1gram of carbohydrates per serving. Their viscous fiber tends to slow down food transport across the digestive tract, encouraging fullness and healthy amounts of blood sugar.

Olives

Olives have, just in strong shape, the same health benefits as olive oil. Olives are high in antioxidants, which may help improve the protection of the heart and bones. They produce 1gram per ounce of net carbohydrates.

Unsweetened Coffee and Tea

Coffee and tea are unbelievably healthy drinks that are carb-free. Unsweetened coffee and tea do not contain carbohydrates and help increase your metabolic rate and physical and mental performance. They will decrease the chance of diabetes as well.

Dark Chocolate and Cocoa Powder

Delicious forms of antioxidants include dark chocolate and cocoa. Dark chocolate is rich in antioxidants, produces 3-10grams of net carbs per ounce, and can significantly minimize heart disease risk.

The Bottom Line

A Ketogenic diet may be used to accomplish weight reduction, blood sugar management, and other health-related targets.

Fortunately, a wide variety of healthy, tasty, and flexible foods that help you stay within your regular carb variety can be found.

Consume all 16 ingredients daily to enjoy all the nutritional advantages of a Ketogenic diet.

What Foods Are Not on the Eating List of Keto?

- Sugar: the most important thing to cut

- Alcohol: too many sugars and carbs

- Fruit: a negligible amount of fruit is right, but adds sugar to your meal

- Starches: white bread, rice, potatoes, pasta

Keto-fying Your Preferred Foods

Any of your favorite foods might be on the list above, based on what you enjoy eating.

It is still difficult to follow the constraints of an alternative lifestyle.

For our friends and us, recipes and food may become so unique that it's impossible to step away from them.

Fortunately, there are convenient ways to produce substitutes for your preferred items, so they work into keto or keep inside a close window, at least.

This means you can always get your pasta dishes and sandwiches in abundance! Pick carbohydrates that are more effective for a low glycemic index.

- Bread: 20x fewer carbs than ordinary bread

- Rice: 3-ingredient recipe

- Pasta: 2-ingredient recipe

- Oatmeal: low-carb breakfast choice

The Best Keto Diets for Women Over 50 to Fulfill Their Health Needs

Their bodies brace for and go through menopause and other side effects of aging as women reach 50. To improve their wellbeing, many women need to follow new and varied methods, including changing their diets to get the required nutrients. In any scenario, women over 50 may want to check on the right diets.

Thanks to perimenopause and menopause, the 50s was a period for major adjustments. This is a phase in a woman's life when she has variations of hormones, which can trigger metabolism and body weight shifts. Besides, osteoporosis, osteoarthritis, and improvements in blood sugar control (insulin resistance may occur because of hormone adjustments) can arise when people can develop other disorders in this age group.

To help respond to normal shifts in their bodies, women should change their diets. For women over 50 who will help foster good body density, hormonal regulation, and weight control, below are the perfect foods, or rather, lifestyles.

Mediterranean

For cardiac wellbeing, the Mediterranean diet is perfect and will avoid cancer and diabetes. It does not exclude or exclude certain food types but supports all in balance instead. Compared to whole grains, which contain a lot of fiber and can keep you feeling satisfied for longer, it stresses carbs from fruits and vegetables.

Omega-3 fats that are present in seafood and olive oil are illustrated in the Mediterranean diet. Besides helping with hormone production, it has plenty of omega-3 fats found in fish and olive oil, enhancing satiety. It's also rich in nutrition, both in goods dependent on plants and livestock. For women over 50 who need it to combat muscle loss that develops with age, this protein is important.

Paleo

A high-protein, low-calorie meal plan heavy in eggs, plants, citrus, nuts, and unprocessed meat is the Paleo diet. For women in their 50s and older who might struggle with insulin resistance and cannot handle carbohydrates as they were before, the lower carbohydrate existence is helpful.

The Pale diet stresses protein and soy and dairy are reduced. Paleo does not include soy or beef and may support people with hormonal shifts since extra soy and hormones present in traditional dairy goods may contribute to elevated estrogen levels, causing people to store weight in their thighs and hips. Good fats that encourage the safe development of hormones are also included.

Whole Foods

The entire diet for organic food, or "good eating," eliminates any processed items that may reduce inflammation. Thanks to the fact that whole foods do not contain pesticides or preservatives, which can be major hormone disruptors, this diet may also help regulate hormones.

On the Whole Foods diet, processed foods are not required. It emphasizes all authentic food items, such as fruits, herbs, legumes, whole grains, seafood, beef, and balanced fats. Few added carbohydrates are equivalent to the absence of processed food, resulting in greater blood sugar stability and less belly fat being kept. In these ingredients, the high volume of nutrients and fiber often contributes to feeling whole, avoiding overeating.

Autoimmune Protocol (AIP)

The Autoimmune Protocol (AIP) focuses on intestinal recovery and reducing inflammation and may benefit people with hormonal shifts in their 50s. It may also eliminate harmful substances and activate substances that can induce mal-absorption and inflammation in the stomach, such as refined sugars and packaged foods.

It prevents the capacity of the body to consume nutrients if the gut is toxic. This induces hormonal imbalances that worsen the shifts in hormones that are already taking place. AIP also helps the immune system, which, when we mature, will reduce the likelihood of infection.

Higher Protein/Moderate Carbohydrate

The body can be assisted through its normal aging period by consuming a high protein/ moderate carbohydrate diet. Studies also showed that higher amounts of protein help the body's muscle mass, and it reduces when you mature and therefore holds you whole, lowering the amount of food eaten.

6. BAD EATING HABITS WILL NOT IMPROVE YOUR HEALTH

Selecting the right food option is one of the major challenges people above 50 have to face in Keto. According to their age bracket, it is difficult for them to adjust their meal options. Not all people are flexible enough to shift their food preference to 180 degrees or 360 degrees at this age. It can be difficult, but not impossible. A little effort can help them have better food options. You can find out more guidelines about this in later chapters.

Managing Health Issues:

The Keto diet solves many of your health problems. It helps people above the age of 50 deal with many developing and lifelong health problems or issues. On the other hand, it is necessary to manage these problems with a diet plan in the beginning. Many people suffering from specific diet-based problems, such as blood pressure, hypertension, diabetes, and more, must take care of multiple things. Lately, they will manage and test the proper solution to these issues and problems.

Avoiding Additional Risks

Another important challenge of the Keto diet is to ensure you will not face some other crucial problems. It happens if you follow any diet plan blindly and do not focus on the important things. Here, you may have to face other problems as well. It is necessary to manage everything in the beginning so you can avoid any further risk.

Controlling Cravings

Food cravings are one of the major challenges in all kinds of diet plans. When you have a specification of not eating something, you urge to consume that specific thing, for sure. Your brain plays a major role in the trigger of these things. For the people above 50, it is often difficult to control cravings because of habit. In the 50 years of life, consuming specific food items seems to be a habit. It is necessary to find out their alternative and pick up the options to avoid such problems and matters. It is not difficult to deceive these cravings; all you need is proper research and homework.

Dealing with Reactions

Most of the time, Keto comes up with several reactions and changes in the body. It is obvious when you make some visible changes to your overall food intake. Then you will have to face changes in the body. In this scenario, it is important to deal with things appropriately. It is a suggestion to have a dietitian or nutritionist to consult so you can manage these things.

On the other hand, you need to have prior information about the possible reactions. It will help you to deal with them with time. Moreover, you can adopt some of the precautions that help you to avoid these things moving forward. In the next chapters, you will know about the major reactions and complications that can hit an above 50 Keto followers.

In a Ketogenic diet, a person has to cut the one major food group from their diet—carbohydrates that help build muscles, grow, and provide strength. To manage the intake from the substitute option, it is necessary to understand the possible deficiencies that a person can face due to keto.

Here are some necessary nutrients that the body requires for effective body functioning:

Sodium

Sodium is considered an important element for the body, and, due to the keto diet, it is possible to lose the optimal amount from the body. Due to a low carb diet, a person has to resist salt consumption and other carbohydrates. Moreover, due to ketosis, the body consumes sodium as an electrolyte that causes a reduction in the sodium element. It affects daily activities and energy levels, as well. To overcome the issue, you can add some salt to your meal per the daily calorie count details.

Potassium

With the sodium reduction, the body starts losing potassium as well. It can weaken the muscles and cause constipation and other irritability in the body. To overcome the potassium deficiency, a person can use the low carbs food options like mushrooms, avocado, kale or spinach in their meal—they are high in potassium and reduce fatigue and cognitive issues.

Magnesium

Magnesium deficiency can cause muscle cramps, dizziness, and nausea and affect the reproduction of the cells and tissues in the body. In the body, there are multiple chemical processes in which magnesium is a vital element. It is important to overcome the possible deficiency of the element in a Ketogenic diet, which can be overcome by adding seeds into the diet, like pumpkin seeds, etc. Spinach is also a great source to overcome magnesium deficiency in keto.

Calcium

Calcium plays an important role in bone growth, strength and is also good for cognitive efficiency. In the process of ketosis, the chances of calcium deficiency become higher. It is the one major element that the body will lose during the Ketogenic diet. To regain and maintain the body's optimal level, consume almonds, nuts, broccoli, and add cheese and fish in the keto meals.

Vitamins

Vitamins are micronutrients that are important for body functions. They also play an important role in muscle building, fat reduction, and multiple other body functions. Vegetables, especially green leafy ones, offer many vitamins for those on the keto diet. Meat, nuts, and dairy items like cheese can be consumed as sources to add enough vitamins to the diet.

The Most Common Mistakes to Try to Lose Weight

Even if you reach your 50s, that doesn't mean that you can't make a mistake, especially when starting something new like the Ketogenic diet. A lot of beginners, irrespective of age, make the same mistakes when following the low-carb diet. Check out the list of the top mistakes people often make and avoid them if you want to get brilliant results from such an effective diet.

- Inadequate Fluid Intake. On a keto diet, the body tries to burn more fat, and that's why it needs to be well-hydrated. Most people focus just on what they're eating and forget about what they're sipping. This mistake leads to a slower metabolism and, thus, halting weight-shedding. Besides, water is essential for nutrient circulation and flushing out toxins. So, if you're going to fasten your ketosis and improve your health, try to consume 3-4 liters of water (or even more) per day.

- Dairy Over-Enrichment. Remember, moderation is the key for you. Of course, you may find that dairy products are great for the Keto dieting plan. They're ideal high fat and low-carb sources. However, don't forget that some dairy products contain sugar and overeating them can destroy your dieting plan. Because of this, you need to calculate the dairy products' calories and pay attention to their nutrition labels.

- Lack of Fat. For the Keto diet it means a low-carb and high-fat intake. At least 75% of the calories you consume should be provided from animal fats, monounsaturated fats, and olive oil. In such away, you can ensure normal hormone function and boost your metabolism.

- Excess Protein Intake. We've drawn attention to the fact that if you eat too much protein, it'll cause adverse effects. Excess protein will be converted into glucose by your body, and this can ruin your dietary needs.

- Not Preparing Yourself for 'Fat Adaptation.' It can be a bit time-consuming for your body to get used to burning off fat instead of glucose for fuel. So, prepare yourself and your body to experience the 'Fat Adaptation' or 'Keto Flu.' During the first week and even the second one, you may feel more tired, aches, and muscle cramps. That's pretty normal when your body adapts to another dietary need.

- Concealment from Your doctor. Think about your age... Your doctor has the right to know about every change in your life. And especially for nutritional changes. Talk to your doctor before including Keto products in your diet plan to ensure that this's a good idea for you, and it won't harm your health.

7. FOODS YOU SHOULD EAT AND FOODS TO AVOID

The Ketogenic diet is high in fats, moderate in proteins, and low in carbs. For a person to reach ketosis naturally in the body, the body consumes fast to get the energy in the absence of carbs. According to studies, it is proven to be an effective and result-oriented way to lose weight and have a healthy lifestyle.

Before starting following the diet, a person has to understand: what is it all about? This includes what you can eat or what you should avoid in the whole procedure. The primary purpose of keto is to restrict the number of carbs, because it is a source of glucose and other components that can slow down weight loss.

What Should You Eat in the Ketogenic Diet?

For those people who follow the Ketogenic diet to lose weight, it is important to follow the high fats or protein options and restrict the number of carbs. First, only 5% of carbs are allowed to be consumed from a meal in a day. Similarly, 20% of the proteins can be added. The portion, around 70% to 80%, must be fat.

Food to Have as Carbs

To fulfill the 5% carbs requirement, it is necessary to go with the right choice. Here is the list of the food items that are completely keto-friendly and offer the carbs necessary to have in a Ketogenic diet plan:

- Tomato

- Broccoli

- Spinach

- Bell pepper

- Cucumber

- Celery

- Zucchini

- Brussels sprout

- Cauliflower
- Asparagus
- Kale

Food to Have as Proteins

Proteins are good to have in the meal and rich in sources to fuel up the body. Moreover, it offers the muscles strength and plays a role in building cells and tissues. Here are options that you can add as a protein in your keto meal:

- Chicken
- Lamb
- Beef
- Salmon
- Eggs
- Organic cheese
- Whole milk cheese
- Shrimp
- Greek yogurt

Food to Have as Fats

In the Ketogenic diet, fat is important, and the major component that has to be maximum in quantity to put the body in ketosis. But while choosing the options, be sure to pick the healthy fats instead of non-organic fat options. Here are some options that you can add as good fats in your meal:

- Nuts
- Seeds
- Avocado
- Olive oil
- Avocado oil
- Cheese
- Cream cheese
- Heavy cream
- Coconuts
- Flaxseeds

- Peanut butter

- Sesame seeds

- Pumpkin seeds

- Olives

- Butter, etc.

What Should You Avoid in a Ketogenic Diet?

In the keto diet, an individual should avoid high carbs and starchy food. Because it can reduce the process of fats reduction, and you cannot get the proper health benefit of the following keto. Here is a list of foods you should avoid during the keto diet:

- Rice, pasta, oatmeal and grains

- Low-fat dairy items

- Sweeteners and added sugar

- Beverages, drinks and juices, whether natural or canned

- Avoid snacks, crackers and chips, etc.

- Starchy vegetables like potatoes, corn and peas

- Non-organic fats like kinds of margarine, etc.

Planning Your Mealtime

The most difficult thing in managing the keto diet is preparing for the meal. To get the real benefits out of the diet plan, it is important to cook your food by yourself instead of going to the prepared one. But most people complain that with a busy schedule, it is complicated to follow the pattern diet. To get the maximum advantage, it is important to prepare a schedule and dedicate each meal a time.

To avoid the hassle and avail the healthy and keto-friendly options to eat, prepare and store meals for later use. You can get multiple recipe ideas to prepare on weekends and enjoy for the entire week, even with a tough schedule. While preparing the meal and planning the time, it is important to consider the keto diet's basic rules—low carbs, high fats, and proteins. Check the nutrients of the food group you are taking as the meal option.

According to a study, a person can take up to nine meals in a keto diet throughout the day. But the concern is that all should be segregated according to the right blend of macros. To start and keep yourself fit on the plan, you can get the help of a keto meter. This helps to record the macros. Use the right percentage to get the most benefits. Plan a 30-day meal plan and segregate each week separately with the designated meal option for breakfast, lunch, dinner, and snacks.

At the start, it is really difficult to avoid the cravings and be strict with the low carbs meal options. Thanks to the Ketogenic meal options, you can try traditional things but in a different and low carb style. So, now you do not need to sacrifice your favorite food and have one with balanced ingredients.

The Things to Keep in Mind as a Senior on the Keto Diet

Seniors have some different considerations than other folks who are on the Keto Diet. Because seniors may have other health conditions, they should check with their doctor before going full speed into the Keto Diet. The good thing about the Keto Diet is that there are many benefits for seniors, especially when it comes to the cognitive benefits and lowering the chances of being on the wrong end of neurological disorders such as Parkinson's and Alzheimer's. For seniors, many benefits will improve the quality of life from now on. Having the Keto Diet as part of their way of life will make sure they are in the best position to take care of their health.

One thing that seniors should pay attention to is how they are feeling. Seniors who are experiencing digestive issues that do not resolve should head to the doctor right away. Diarrhea is something that can't be resolved with just drinking more water, same with constipation when it gets to be pervasive. Making sure that the health considerations and any adverse effects are managed is very important.

Another thing to keep in mind that checking the ketone levels is also very important. If a senior is not checking their ketone levels, then what they are doing is not knowing if they are in ketosis or not. This is important. It is the whole point of the diet. Make sure you are in Ketosis by checking your breath, your blood, and your urine.

If you are diabetic or prediabetic, it is imperative to check with your doctor to go on the Keto Diet and navigate through the process. Your doctor will monitor your levels and make sure you do not do something to your body that can cause harm. Communication with your doctor is vitally important to ensure that you get the most out of Keto Diet.

Exercise is something that should be part of the Keto Diet. For seniors, it is not about recapturing their glory days from the youth, but engaging in a physical activity that burns calories and having those calories burn fat cells. Some simple things to do, like walking or bike riding, will give seniors the exercise and stimulation they need to get the most out of their diet. When taking all of these things into consideration, the Keto Diet will be a net positive for seniors.

8. MEAL PLAN AND SHOPPING LIST

You have already learned the nuts and bolts of the keto plan, how and why it is especially helpful for women fifty and older, and how it helps you eat well every day, lose weight, and support your overall good health. You know the foods that are best for you to eat and best to avoid. And you have a wide variety of recipes in your toolbox.

Now you might be looking at all of this information and wondering where to begin. This chapter will get you off to the best possible start. Within these pages, you'll find a 30-day keto-friendly meal plan and a shopping list to take to the grocery store with you.

One of the real benefits of the keto diet plan is how flexible it is. Unlike other diet programs that are so rigid that you have no freedom in your daily meal plans, you can customize keto to fit your own needs and preferences best. Use the 30-day plan as a tool to help you, but know you can make any substitutions to allow you to incorporate all your favorites and skip any recipe or meal idea that isn't as appealing to you.

The majority of these recipes serve more than one, so you will probably have leftovers to incorporate into your menu unless you feed several people every meal. You can assemble several meals each week by choosing some of your favorite fats and proteins, like bacon and eggs for breakfast, or a chicken breast with broccoli for lunch, or a grilled steak with sliced avocado and roasted cauliflower for dinner.

Be creative and piece your meals together in a way that delights you. And know that this 30-day meal plan can help fill in the pieces and provide guidance when you're looking for ideas.

Shopping List

Now that you've got a sample menu, it's time to think about that first trip to the grocery store.

The list provided here is detailed, but you won't need every item, every time.

Use the shopping list below as a general guide for staples that most people on keto find helpful to have on hand. Of course, you will mark off the things you don't find appealing and add specific items for the recipes you want to try.

Return to the early pages of this book and make a note of all the keto-friendly foods that you most enjoy; that's the best place to start. Then, make a note of any ingredients you would need for the recipes in this book you are planning to make first. That will give you a jump-start on the first week or two.

Here is one final note about the recipes and the shopping list. You'll recall reading earlier in the book that choosing whole foods as much as possible is ideal, and choosing highly processed foods should be an occasional addition to your diet, not your entire diet. Things like pepperoni, sausage, and ham show up in some recipes and on the shopping list. Enjoy those things in moderation.

The same is principle holds with certain fruits and vegetables with carbs, like tomatoes, for example. Having a few tomatoes here and there won't derail your plan and keep you from ketosis. Remember, your goal is to consume less than 20grams of carbs per day, so if tomatoes have about 3grams of net carbs per serving, you'll want to be aware and pay attention to your total carb consumption.

Here is one helpful rule of thumb for shopping. For the most part, you'll find the items most beneficial to your foundation of healthy eating around the grocery store's outer edges. The produce section, meat section, seafood section, and dairy section are typically around the store's perimeter. The highly processed foods like cereal, bread, canned goods, chips, sodas, candy, and boxed meal kits are usually on the interior aisles. Fill up on all the things around the outside aisles before going straight to the stuff in the middle you'll need. That will significantly reduce the temptation to smuggle home some of those junk food items.

General Grocery Shopping List for Keto Diet

Center Aisles

- Almond Flour
- Avocado Oil
- Beef Broth
- Chia Seeds
- Chicken Broth
- Cocoa Powder (non-sweetened)
- Coconut Flour
- Coconut Milk
- Coconut Oil
- Dill Pickles
- Flax Seeds
- Green Olives
- Hot Sauce
- Mayonnaise
- Mustard
- Spices and Seasonings

Dairy

- Butter
- Cheese
- Cottage Cheese (full fat)
- Cream
- Cream Cheese
- Eggs
- Greek Yogurt (plain, full fat)
- Heavy Cream
- Parmesan Cheese
- Ricotta Cheese
- Sour Cream

Fruits & Vegetables

- Avocado
- Asparagus
- Berries (blueberries, blackberries)
- Blueberries
- Broccoli
- Brussels Sprouts
- Cabbage
- Cauliflower
- Celery
- Chiles
- Cucumber
- Eggplant
- Green Beans
- Lemons
- Lettuce
- Limes
- Mushrooms
- Onions
- Olives
- Peas
- Peppers
- Squash
- Spinach
- Strawberries
- Tomato
- Zucchini

Meat

- Bacon
- Beef
- Bison
- Chicken
- Duck
- Ham
- Hamburger
- Jerky
- Lamb
- Pepperoni
- Pork
- Sausage
- Steak Turkey

Nuts & Seeds

- Almonds
- Almond Butter
- Brazil Nuts
- Peanuts
- Peanut Butter (watch sugar/carb counts)
- Pecans
- Pumpkin Seeds
- Pistachios
- Sunflower Seeds
- Walnuts

Seafood

- Calamari/Squid
- Crab
- Fish
- Lobster
- Prawns
- Scallops
- Shrimp

9. BREAKFAST

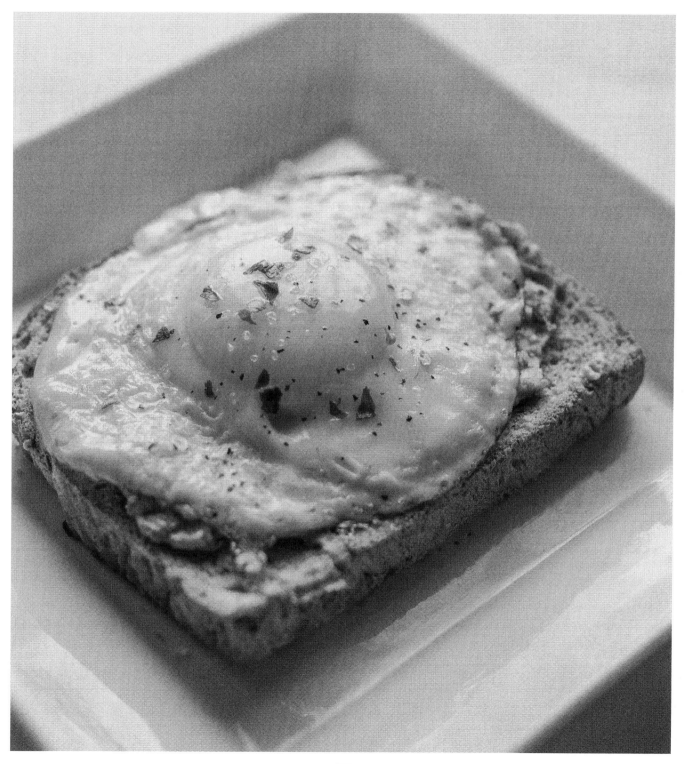

PREPARATION: 10 MIN

COOKING: 12 MIN

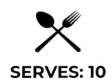
SERVES: 10

ALMOND FLOUR KETO PANCAKES

INGREDIENTS

- 4 oz. softened cream cheese, at room temperature
- Zest of 1 medium-sized lemon, fresh (approximately 1 teaspoon)
- 4 large-sized eggs, organic
- ½ cup almond flour
- 1 tablespoon butter for frying and serving

DIRECTIONS

1. Combine the almond flour with eggs, cream cheese, and lemon zest using a whisk in a medium-sized mixing bowl until combined well and completely smooth, for a minute or two.
2. The next step is to heat a large, nonstick skillet over medium heat until hot. Once done; add 1 tablespoon of butter until completely melted; swirl to coat the bottom completely.
3. Pour 3 tablespoons of the prepared batter (for each pancake) and cook for a minute or two until it turns golden. Carefully flip; cook the other side for 2 more minutes. Transfer to a clean, large plate and continue cooking with the remaining batter.
4. Top the cooked pancakes with some butter; serve immediately and enjoy.

NUTRITION

- Calories: 120
- Total Fat: 8.6g
- Saturated Fat: 3.1g
- Total Carbohydrates: 2g
- Dietary Fiber: 1g
- Sugars: 0.8g
- Protein: 3.9g

PREPARATION: 5 MIN

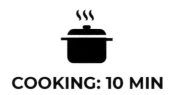
COOKING: 10 MIN

SERVES: 2

KETO COCONUT FLOUR EGG MUFFIN

INGREDIENTS

- 1 organic egg, large-sized
- 2 teaspoons coconut flour or as required
- A pinch of baking soda
- 1 tablespoon coconut oil to coat
- Salt, to taste

DIRECTIONS

1. Preheat your oven to 400°F. Lightly coat a large-sized coffee mug or ramekin dish with some coconut oil.
2. Using a fork, mix the real ingredients and make sure no lumps remain.
3. Bake for 10 to 12 minutes, until cooked through.
4. Cut in half; serve immediately and enjoy.

NUTRITION

- Calories: 48
- Total Fat: 3.9g
- Saturated Fat: 1.1g
- Total Carbohydrates: 1.7g
- Dietary Fiber: 0.3g
- Sugars: 0.5g
- Protein: 3.7g

PREPARATION: 10 MIN

COOKING: 15 MIN

SERVES: 6

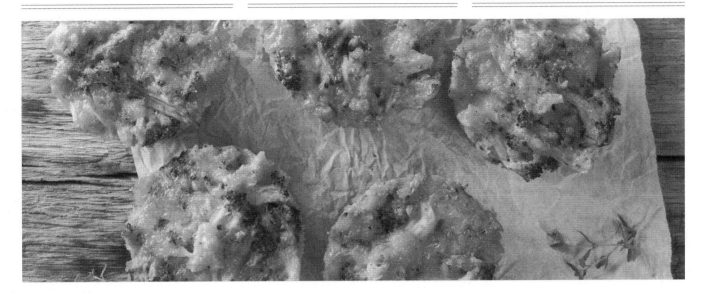

BROCCOLI CHEDDAR CHEESE MUFFINS

INGREDIENTS

- 2/3 cup cheddar cheese, grated plus more for topping
- ¼ teaspoon garlic powder
- ¾ cup broccoli, steamed and chopped (fresh or frozen and thawed)
- ¼ teaspoon dried thyme

DIRECTIONS

1. Preheat your oven to 400°F. Combine the thyme with garlic powder in a large-sized mixing bowl until combined well, and then stir in the cheddar and broccoli. Evenly divide the mixture into the muffin tins (with 6 cups), filling each cup approximately 2/3 full.
2. Sprinkle with more cheddar on top, if desired, and then bake until completely set, for 12 to 15 minutes. Serve immediately and enjoy.

NUTRITION

- Calories: 33
- Total Fat: 4.2g
- Saturated Fat: 2.2g
- Total Carbohydrates: 1.8g
- Dietary Fiber: 0.7g
- Sugars: 0.3g
- Protein: 2.2g

PREPARATION: 10 MIN

COOKING: 0 MIN

SERVES: 4

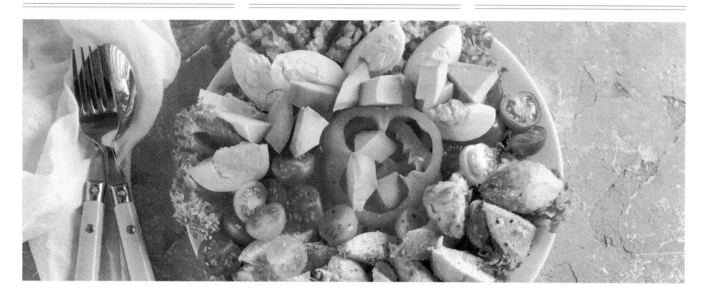

CHICKEN, BACON, AVOCADO CAESAR SALAD

INGREDIENTS

- 1 chicken breast, pre-cooked or grilled, sliced into small bite-sized slices
- 1 avocado, ripe, sliced in half, twist and discard the pit, remove the shell and slice into approximately 1" slices.
- Creamy Caesar dressing (approximately 3 tablespoons per salad)
- 1 cup bacon, pre-cooked, crumbled

DIRECTIONS

1. Combine the chicken breast with avocado slices and crumbled bacon between two large-sized bowls.
2. Top with a few spoonful's of the Creamy Caesar dressing; lightly toss the ingredients.
3. Serve immediately and enjoy.

NUTRITION

- Calories: 322
- Total Fat: 30g
- Saturated Fat: 8.6g
- Total Carbohydrates: 5g
- Dietary Fiber: 3.4g
- Sugars: 0.9g
- Protein: 9.2g

PREPARATION: 15 MIN

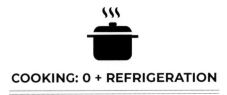
COOKING: 0 + REFRIGERATION

SERVES: 6

COCONUT MACADAMIA BARS

INGREDIENTS

- ½ cup macadamia nuts
- 6 tablespoons unsweetened coconut, shredded
- ½ cup almond butter
- 20 drops of stevia drops, preferably Sweet leaf
- ¼ cup of coconut oil

DIRECTIONS

1. Crush the macadamia nuts using hands or in a food processor.
2. Combine coconut oil with the shredded coconut and almond butter in a large-sized mixing bowl. Add the stevia drops and chopped macadamia nuts.
3. Thoroughly mix and pour the prepared batter into a 9x9" baking dish lined with parchment paper.
4. Refrigerate overnight; slice into desired pieces. Serve and enjoy.

NUTRITION

- Calories: 324
- Total Fat: 32g
- Saturated Fat: 13g
- Total Carbohydrates: 5g
- Dietary Fiber: 4g
- Sugars: 1.8g
- Protein: 5.6g

PREPARATION: 15 MIN

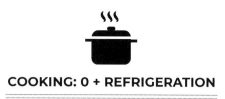

COOKING: 0 + REFRIGERATION

SERVES: 6

MACADAMIA CHOCOLATE FAT BOMB

INGREDIENTS

- 2 oz. Cocoa butter
- 4 oz. macadamias chopped
- 2 tablespoons Swerve
- ¼ cup coconut oil or heavy cream
- 2 tablespoons cocoa powder, unsweetened

DIRECTIONS

1. Fill a large saucepan half full with boiling water. Place a small-sized saucepan over the large saucepan with the boiling water and melt the cocoa butter in it.
2. Once melted, add in the cocoa powder and then add the Swerve; mix well until the real ingredients are completely melted and well blended.
3. Add in the macadamias; give everything a good stir.
4. Now, add the cream or coconut oil; mix well (bringing it to the temperature again). Pour the prepared mixture into paper candy cups or molds, filling them evenly. Let cool for a couple of minutes at room temperature, and then place them in a refrigerator. Let chill until harden. Serve and enjoy.

NUTRITION

- Calories: 267
- Total Fat: 28g
- Saturated Fat: 15g
- Total Carbohydrates: 3g
- Dietary Fiber: 2g
- Sugars: 0.9g
- Protein: 3g

PREPARATION: 10 MIN

COOKING: 0 + 50 MIN REFRIGERATION

SERVES: 6

KETO LEMON BREAKFAST FAT BOMBS

INGREDIENTS

- 10 to 15 drops of Stevia extract
- 1 tablespoon lemon extract or lemon zest, organic
- 1 pack coconut butter or creamed coconut (approximately 3.5 oz.), softened
- 1 oz. Extra virgin coconut oil, softened (approximately 1/8 cup)
- A pinch of Himalayan pink salt or sea salt

DIRECTIONS

1. Zest the lemons and ensure that the coconut oil and coconut butter are at room temperature and softened.
2. Combine the real ingredients in a large-sized mixing bowl and ensure the stevia and lemon zest are dispersed.
3. Fill each silicone candy mold or mini muffin paper cup with approximately 1 tablespoon of the prepared coconut mixture and place them on a large-sized tray.
4. Place the tray inside the fridge and let chill until solid, for 40 to 50 minutes.
5. Keep refrigerated until ready to serve. Serve and enjoy.

NUTRITION

- Calories: 184
- Total Fat: 20g
- Saturated Fat: 14g
- Total Carbohydrates: 0.2g
- Dietary Fiber: 0.1g
- Sugars: 0.1g
- Protein: 0.1g

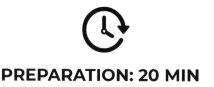

PREPARATION: 20 MIN

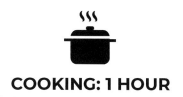

COOKING: 1 HOUR

SERVES: 6

BAKED CUSTARD-DAIRY-FREE

INGREDIENTS

- 3 cups/678g Unsweetened-full-fat coconut milk
- 4 large/200g Raw eggs
- 1 tsp./2.5g Pure vanilla extract, or scrapings from ½ of a vanilla pod
- Optional Sprinkle Topping: Nutmeg/cinnamon
- Also Needed:
- Glass baking dish–to hold serving containers
- 6 oz. glass custard/serving dishes

DIRECTIONS

1. Warm the oven to 350 °Fahrenheit.
2. Boil enough water to come ½ inch from the top of the outside of the custard cups. Place the cups into the pan. (Wait to fill the dish with water.)
3. Whisk the eggs with the milk, sweetener, and vanilla and add it to the cups. Sprinkle cinnamon/nutmeg over the top as desired.
4. Arrange the holding tray on the oven rack and pour the hot water to make the water bath. Bake the custard for 45 minutes.
5. Check for doneness. Insert a knife into the middle of the cup. It's ready if it comes out without custard attached.
6. Carefully transfer the dishes to the countertop or serving tray to serve. Add any leftovers to the fridge with a covering of foil or plastic wrap.

NUTRITION

- Calories: 246
- Net Carbohydrates: 3g
- Protein: 6g

- Fat Content: 24g

PREPARATION: 20 MIN

COOKING: 1 HOUR

SERVES: 6

OLD-FASHIONED BAKED CUSTARD– HEAVY CREAM

INGREDIENTS

- .5 cup Water
- 2.5 cups/565g 36% heavy cream
- 4 large/200g Raw egg
- 1 tsp./2.5g Pure vanilla extract, or Pod scrapings (½ of a vanilla pod)
- Optional Toppings:
- Sweetener–your preference
- Nutmeg or cinnamon
- Also Needed:
- Glass baking dish
- 6 oz. Glass custard dishes

DIRECTIONS

1. Measure and boil water to make a water bath using the baking dish. It needs to be enough to extend three-quarters of the way up the custard cups (fill in the last step).
2. Set the oven to 350° Fahrenheit.
3. Use a mixing container to whisk the eggs with the water, vanilla, cream, and sweetener— if using.
4. Scoop the custard into the serving cups. (Place the cups in the baking dish before you begin.) Sprinkle using a dusting of the nutmeg or cinnamon to your liking.
5. Arrange the baking dish on the oven rack. Pour the hot water into the ½-inch marker of the cups.
6. Set a timer to bake for 45 minutes. It should be firmly set. Test it using a knife in the middle of the custard. If it comes out mostly clean, it's ready.
7. Serve the custard warm. Store it with a covering of foil or plastic in the refrigerator.

NUTRITION

- Calories: 370
- Net Carbohydrates: 3g
- Protein: 6g
- Fat Content: 37g

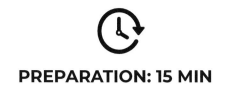
PREPARATION: 15 MIN

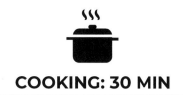
COOKING: 30 MIN

SERVES: 6

BACON & EGG FAT BOMBS

INGREDIENTS

- 4.2 oz. Or 4 large Bacon slices
- 2 Large organic eggs
- .25 cup Ghee or butter
- 1 pinch Black pepper
- .25 tsp Salt
- 2 tbsp Mayonnaise

DIRECTIONS

1. Set the oven temperature at 375° Fahrenheit.
2. Arrange the bacon slices on a parchment paper-lined baking tin. Bake it; / for 10 to 15 minutes. Drain and reserve the grease.
3. On the stovetop, boil the eggs for ten minutes in salted water. Quickly add them into an ice bath to cool. Peel and slice the eggs and add the butter or ghee to the eggs. Smash with a fork.
4. Combine the pepper, salt, mayonnaise, and bacon grease. Stir thoroughly and place it in the refrigerator for 20-30 minutes.
5. Meanwhile, crumble the strips of bacon in a container for breading the bombs. Form six balls using an ice cream scoop for uniform sizing. Roll them in the bits and place them in the fridge.

NUTRITION

- Calories: 185
- Net Carbohydrates: 0.2g
- Protein: 5g

- Fat Content: 18g

PREPARATION: 5 MIN

COOKING: 5 MIN

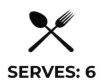

SERVES: 6

BEST SCRAMBLED EGGS

INGREDIENTS

- 4 large Eggs
- Salt and pepper (as desired)
- .25 cup Skim or 1% milk
- 2 tbsp Fresh parsley
- Cooking oil spray (as needed)

DIRECTIONS

1. Finely chop the parsley. Break eggs into a bowl and add the milk, pepper, salt, and parsley. Whisk until thoroughly combined.
2. Warm a skillet using the med-high temperature setting and lightly spritz it using the cooking spray.
3. Pour eggs into the pan, pushing them around the pan with a non-metal spatula until the eggs are set, and no liquid remains (5 min.).
4. Scrape the pan and continue stirring to keep the eggs light.
5. Note: For the best results, don't use egg beaters! They will not properly cook.

NUTRITION

- Calories: 161.5
- Net Carbohydrates: 2.9g
- Protein: 13.7g
- Fat Content: 10.1g

PREPARATION: 3 MIN

COOKING: 4 MIN

SERVES: 6

CREAM CHEESE EGGS

INGREDIENTS

- 1 tbsp Butter
- 2 Eggs
- 2 tbsp Soft cream cheese with chives

DIRECTIONS

1. Heat a skillet and melt the butter. Whisk the eggs with the cream cheese.
2. Add to the pan and serve when ready.

NUTRITION

- Calories: 341
- Net Carbohydrates: 3g
- Protein: 15g

- Fat Content: 29g

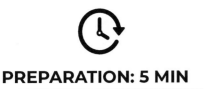

PREPARATION: 5 MIN

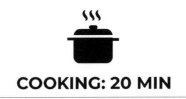

COOKING: 20 MIN

SERVES: 9

HAM & EGG CUPS

INGREDIENTS

- 5 large/250grams Fresh eggs, fresh
- .5 cup/135grams 36% heavy cream
- 7 oz. Pkg.Natural Uncured Black Forest Ham by Applegate
- 5grams/1 tsp. Coconut oil
- Also Needed: Muffin tin (at least 9-count)
- Salt and pepper

DIRECTIONS

1. Set the oven temperature at 425° Fahrenheit. Lightly grease nine wells/cups of a muffin tin with a spritz of cooking oil.
2. Arrange one slice of ham in each of the muffin wells/cups, pressing the ham's slices into the cups centered with the ham covering the sides and bottoms.
3. Whisk and thoroughly combine the cream, egg, pepper, and salt. Fill nine of the muffin cups.
4. Bake until the egg centers have puffed, and the eggs are set (7-10 min). They might slightly jiggle if shaken but shouldn't be runny/liquid.
5. Add desired garnishes such as green onion or roasted red peppers, or feta cheese, but add the extra carbs.

NUTRITION

- Calories: 117
- Net Carbohydrates: 0.96g
- Protein: 7.72g
- Fat Content: 9.17g
- Calories: 117
- Net Carbohydrates: 0.96g
- Protein: 7.72g
- Fat Content: 9.17g

PREPARATION: 5 MIN

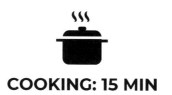

COOKING: 15 MIN

SERVES: 2

HAM & SPINACH MINI QUICHE

INGREDIENTS

- .75 cup Chopped spinach
- .25 cup Chopped leek
- 3 Whisked eggs
- 4 slices Diced ham
- .25 cup Coconut milk
- .5 tspBaking powder
- Pepper & Salt (to taste)
- Also Needed: 4 small quiche or tart pans

DIRECTIONS

1. Set the oven temperature to reach 350° Fahrenheit.
2. Combine all of the fixings in a large mixing container.
3. Empty the mixture into the pans.
4. Bake for 15 minutes. Serve or store for later.

NUTRITION

- Calories: 210
- Net Carbohydrates: 2g
- Protein: 20g
- Fat Content: 13g

PREPARATION: 10 MIN

COOKING: 20 MIN

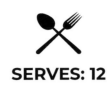
SERVES: 12

SAUSAGE EGG CASSEROLE

INGREDIENTS

- 12 oz. Cooked-browned breakfast sausage-low-fat & reduced-sodium
- 12 large Eggs
- .25 cup Skim milk
- 2 cups Low-fat cheddar cheese (shredded)
- .25 tsp. Black pepper

DIRECTIONS

1. Set the oven to 375° Fahrenheit. Use paper or lightly grease a 12-count muffin pan or grease a casserole dish.
2. Add the batter and bake for ½ hour. Cool for five minutes before serving.

NUTRITION

- Calories: 200.5
- Net Carbohydrates: 2.1g
- Protein: 15.7g
- Fat Content: 39.4g

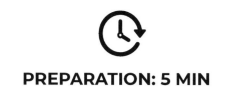

PREPARATION: 5 MIN

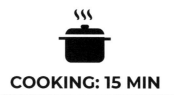

COOKING: 15 MIN

SERVES: 1

SCRAMBLED EGGS WITH MAYO

INGREDIENTS

- 1/50g Large raw egg
- 10g Butter
- 23g Organic mayonnaise–ex. - Trader Joe's
- 1 pinch Salt

DIRECTIONS

1. Prepare a small pan to melt the butter.
2. Whisk the mayo with the egg until thoroughly mixed.
3. Cook and swirl the egg until done. Serve promptly.

NUTRITION

- Calories: 307
- Net Carbohydrates: 0.99g
- Protein: 6.6g
- Fat Content: 30.81g

PREPARATION: 5 MIN

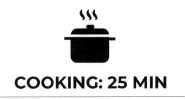

COOKING: 25 MIN

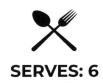

SERVES: 6

BACON & BRIE FRITTATA

INGREDIENTS

- 8 Slices of bacon
- 8 large Eggs
- .5 cup Heavy whipping cream
- 2 Garlic cloves
- .5 tsp. each, Salt and black pepper
- 4 oz. Brie sliced thin (easiest to do when it's cold)
- Also Needed: 10-inch oven-proof skillet

DIRECTIONS

1. Chop and fry the bacon in the skillet using the medium heat temperature setting until it is crispy. Transfer it to drain on a paper towel-lined plate. (Leave at least two to three tablespoons of bacon grease in the skillet and remove from heat). Let the skillet cool.
2. Mince the garlic. Whisk the eggs with the garlic, salt, pepper, cream, and about ⅔ of the cooked bacon. Set the skillet over medium-low heat and swirl the remaining bacon grease to coat its bottom and sides.
3. Add the mix to the skillet (undisturbed) and cook for seven to ten minutes, leaving it somewhat loose to add the bacon's brie and rest.
4. Warm the broiler and place the skillet on the second-highest rack.
5. Broil for about two to five minutes. Remove the pan and cool it for a couple of minutes to serve.

NUTRITION

- Calories: 338
- Net Carbohydrates: 1.7g
- Protein: 18g

- Fat Content: 27g

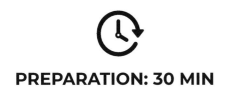
PREPARATION: 30 MIN

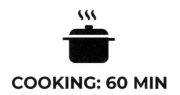
COOKING: 60 MIN

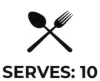
SERVES: 10

JALAPENO POPPERS

INGREDIENTS

- 5 fresh jalapenos, sliced and seeded
- 4 oz. package cream cheese
- ¼ lb. bacon, sliced in half

DIRECTIONS

1. Preheat your oven to 275 degrees F.
2. Place a wire rack over your baking sheet.
3. Stuff each jalapeno with cream cheese and wrap in bacon.
4. Secure with a toothpick.
5. Place on the baking sheet.
6. Bake for 1 hour and 15 minutes.

NUTRITION

- Calories: 103
- Total Fat: 8.7g
- Saturated Fat: 4.1g
- Cholesterol: 25mg
- Sodium: 296mg
- Total Carbohydrate: 0.9g
- Dietary Fiber: 0.2g
- Total Sugars: 0.3g
- Protein: 5.2g
- Potassium: 93mg

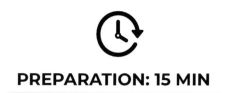
PREPARATION: 15 MIN

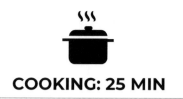
COOKING: 25 MIN

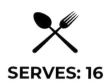
SERVES: 16

EGGS BENEDICT DEVILED EGGS

INGREDIENTS

- 8 hard-boiled eggs, sliced in half
- 1 tablespoon lemon juice
- ½ teaspoon mustard powder
- 1 pack Hollandaise sauce mix, prepared according to a direction in the packaging
- 1 lb. Asparagus, trimmed and steamed
- 4 oz. Bacon, cooked and chopped

DIRECTIONS

1. Scoop out the egg yolks.
2. Mix the egg yolks with lemon juice, mustard powder, and 1/3 cup of the Hollandaise sauce.
3. Spoon the egg yolk mixture into each of the egg whites.
4. Arrange the asparagus spears on a serving plate.
5. Top with the deviled eggs.
6. Sprinkle remaining sauce and bacon on top.

NUTRITION

- Calories: 80
- Total Fat: 5.3g
- Saturated Fat: 1.7g
- Cholesterol: 90mg
- Sodium: 223mg
- Total Carbohydrate: 2.1g
- Dietary Fiber: 0.6g
- Total Sugars: 0.7g
- Protein: 6.2g
- Potassium: 133mg

10. LUNCH

PREPARATION: 5 MIN

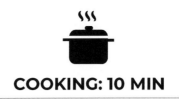
COOKING: 10 MIN

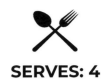
SERVES: 4

CREAM CHEESE STUFFED BABY PEPPERS

INGREDIENTS

- 6 Organic baby peppers
- 6 tablespoons Cream cheese, full-fat

DIRECTIONS

1. Rinse peppers, pat dry with paper towels, then slice the top off.
2. Remove seeds from each pepper, then stuff with cream cheese until full.
3. Serve immediately

NUTRITION

- Calories: 145
- Fat: 12g
- Protein: 3.7g

- Net Carbs: 6.7g
- Fiber: 1g

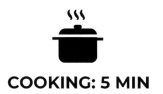
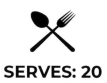
ARTICHOKE DIP

INGREDIENTS

- 10 ounce Frozen spinach
- 14 ounce Artichoke hearts, chopped
- 3 garlic cloves, peeled
- 1 teaspoon Onion powder
- ½ cup Mayonnaise, full-fat
- 12 ounces Parmesan cheese, grated and full-fat
- 8 ounces Cream cheese, full-fat
- ½ cup Sour cream, full-fat
- 12 ounces Swiss cheese, grated, full-fat
- ½ cup Chicken broth, organic

DIRECTIONS

1. Switch on an instant pot, place all the ingredients except for Swiss cheese and parmesan cheese, and stir until mixed.
2. Shut an instant pot with its lid, sealed completely, press the manual button and cook eggs for 4 minutes at high pressure.
3. When done, let the pressure release naturally for 5 minutes, then do quick pressure release and open the instant pot.
4. Add Swiss and parmesan cheese into the instant pot and stir well until cheeses melt and are well combined.
5. Serve immediately.

NUTRITION

- Calories: 230.7
- Fat: 18.7g
- Protein: 12.6g

- Net Carbs: 2.6g
- Fiber: 0.7g

PREPARATION: 5 MIN

COOKING: 8 MIN

SERVES: 8

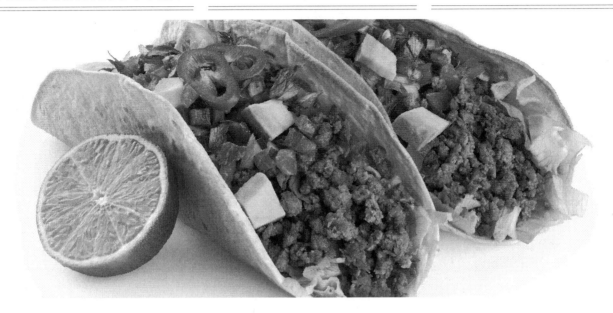

TACO MEAT

INGREDIENTS

- 2 pound Ground turkey
- ½ cup Diced white onion
- ½ cup Diced red bell pepper
- 1 cup Tomato sauce, unsalted
- 1 ½ tablespoon Taco seasoning
- 1 ½ tablespoon Fajita seasoning
- 1 teaspoon Avocado oil
- Avocado slices
- Cilantro

DIRECTIONS

1. Switch on the instant pot, grease pot with oil, press the 'sauté/simmer' button, wait until the oil is hot, and add the ground turkey and cook for 7 to 10 minutes or until nicely browned.
2. Then add remaining ingredients, stir until mixed and press the 'keep warm' button.
3. Shut the instant pot with its lid in the sealed position, press the 'manual' button, press '+/-' to set the cooking time to 8 minutes, and cook at a high-pressure setting pressure builds in the pot. The cooking timer will start.
4. When the instant pot buzzes, press the 'keep warm' button, do a quick pressure release and open the lid.
5. Transfer taco meat to a bowl, top with avocado slices, garnish with cilantro and serve.

NUTRITION

- Calories: 231
- Fat: 14g
- Protein: 21g
- Net Carbs: 2.5g
- Fiber: 1.5g

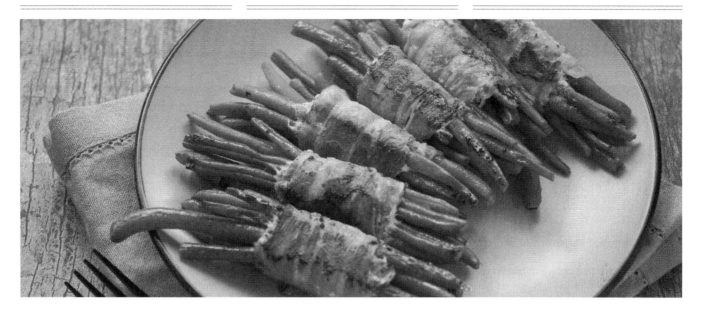

GREEN BEANS WITH BACON

INGREDIENTS

- 5 Slices of bacon chopped
- 6 cups Green beans halved
- 1 teaspoon Salt
- 1 teaspoon Ground black pepper
- ¼ cup Water
- 2 tablespoons Avocado oil

DIRECTIONS

1. Switch on the instant pot, place all the ingredients in it except for oil, and stir until mixed.
2. Shut the instant pot with its lid in the sealed position, press the 'manual' button, press '+/-' to set the cooking time to 4 minutes, and cook at a high-pressure setting pressure builds in the pot. The cooking timer will start.
3. When the instant pot buzzes, press the 'keep warm' button, do a quick pressure release and open the lid.
4. Transfer the greens and bacon to a dish, drizzle with oil, toss until well coated and serve.

NUTRITION

- Calories: 153
- Fat: 9.2g
- Protein: 7g

- Net Carbs: 4.4g
- Fiber: 5.6g

PREPARATION: 5 MIN

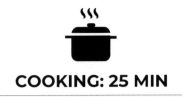
COOKING: 25 MIN

SERVES: 4

BEEF AND BROCCOLI

INGREDIENTS

- 1 ½ pound Chuck roast, sliced
- 12 ounces Broccoli florets
- 4 Garlic cloves peeled
- 2 tablespoons Avocado oil
- ½ cup Soy sauce
- ¼ cup Erythritol sweetener
- 1 tablespoon Xanthan gum

DIRECTIONS

1. Switch on the instant pot, grease the pot with oil, press the 'sauté/simmer' button, wait until the oil is hot and add the beef slices and garlic and cook for 5 to 10 minutes or until browned.
2. Meanwhile, whisk together sweetener, soy sauce, and broth until combined.
3. Pour sauce over browned beef, toss until well coated, press the 'keep warm' button and shut the instant pot with its lid in the sealed position.
4. Press the 'manual' button, press '+/-' to set the cooking time to 10 minutes and cook at a high-pressure setting; when the pressure builds in the pot, the cooking timer will start.
5. Meanwhile, place broccoli florets in a large heatproof bowl, cover with plastic wrap and microwave for 4 minutes or until tender.
6. When the instant pot buzzes, press the 'keep warm' button, do a quick pressure release and open the lid.
7. Take out ¼ cup of cooking liquid, stir in xanthan gum until combined, then add into the instant pot and stir until mixed.
8. Press the 'sauté/simmer' button and simmer beef and sauce for 5 minutes or until the sauce reaches the desired consistency.
9. Then add broccoli florets, stir until mixed and press the cancel button.
10. Serve broccoli and beef with cauliflower rice.

NUTRITION

- Calories: 351.4
- Fat: 12.4g
- Protein: 29g
- Net Carbs: 11g
- Fiber: 8g

PREPARATION: 5 MIN

COOKING: 3 MIN

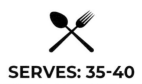

SERVES: 35-40

MEATBALLS

INGREDIENTS

- 1 1/4 pounds Ground beef, pastured
- 1/2 Medium white onion, peeled, minced
- 1 tablespoon Minced garlic
- 1/2 teaspoon Ground black pepper
- 1 teaspoon Salt
- 1 teaspoon Crushed red pepper flakes
- 1/4 cup Fresh rosemary, chopped
- 2 tablespoons Butter, grass-fed, unsalted, softened
- 1 tablespoon Apple cider vinegar

DIRECTIONS

1. Set oven to 350 degrees F and let preheat until meatballs are ready to bake.
2. Place all the ingredients in a bowl, stir until well combined, shape the mixture into meatballs, 1 tablespoon per meatball, and place them on a baking tray lined with parchment sheets.
3. Place the baking tray into the oven and bake the meatballs for 20 minutes or until thoroughly cooked and nicely golden brown.
4. When done, cool the meatballs, place them in batches in the meal prep glass containers and refrigerate for up to 5 days or freeze for up to 3 months.
5. When ready to serve, reheat the meatballs in the oven at 400 degrees F for 7 to 10 minutes or until hot.
6. Serve meatballs with zucchini noodles.

NUTRITION

- Calories: 474
- Fat: 21.7g
- Protein: 61.3g
- Net Carbs: 3.1g
- Fiber: 2.5g

PREPARATION: 10 MIN

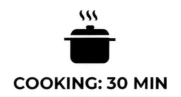
COOKING: 30 MIN

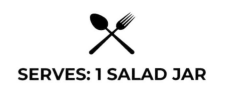
SERVES: 1 SALAD JAR

RAINBOW MASON JAR SALAD

INGREDIENTS

- For the Salad:
- 1/2 cup Arugula, fresh
- 2 Medium radishes, sliced
- 1/4 Medium yellow squash, spiralizer
- 1/4 cup Butternut squash, peeled, cubed
- 1/4 cup Fresh blueberries
- 1 tablespoon Avocado oil
- The Dressing:
- 1/4 Medium avocado, peeled, cubed
- 2 tablespoons Avocado oil
- 1 tablespoon Apple cider vinegar
- 1 tablespoon Filtered water
- 1 tablespoon Cilantro leaves
- 1/4 teaspoon Salt

DIRECTIONS

1. Set oven to 350 degrees F and let preheat.
2. Then place cubes of butternut squash in a bowl, drizzle with oil, toss until well coated, and dispersed on a baking sheet.
3. Place the baking sheet into the oven and bake for 30 minutes or until tender.
4. Meanwhile, prepare the salad dressing and for this, place all the ingredients for the dressing in a blender and pulse for 1 to 2 minutes or until smooth, set aside until required.
5. When the butternut squash is baked, take out the oven's baking sheet and let the squash cool for 15 minutes.
6. Then take a 32-ounce mason jar, pour in the prepared dressing, layer with radish, and top with roasted butternut squash, squash noodles, berries, and arugula.
7. Seal the jar and store in the refrigerator for up to 5 days.

NUTRITION

- Calories: 516
- Fat: 49g
- Protein: 2g
- Net Carbs: 6g
- Fiber: 6g

PREPARATION: 10 MIN

COOKING: 8 MIN

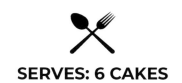
SERVES: 6 CAKES

FISH CAKES

INGREDIENTS

- For Fish Cakes:
- 1 pound Whitefish fillet, wild-caught
- 1/4 cup Cilantro leaves and stem
- ¼ teaspoon Salt
- 1/8 teaspoon Red chili flakes
- 2 Garlic cloves, peeled
- 2 tablespoons Avocado oil
- Dipping Sauce:
- 2 Avocados, peeled, pitted
- 1 Lemon, juiced
- 1/8 teaspoon Salt
- 2 tablespoons Water

DIRECTIONS

1. Prepare the fish cakes and for this, place all the ingredients for the cake in a food processor, except for oil, and pulse for 1 to 2 minutes until evenly combined.
2. Then take a large skillet pan, place it on medium-high heat, add oil and leave until hot.
3. Shape the fish cake mixture into six patties, add them into the heated pan in a single layer and cook for 4 minutes per side or until thoroughly cooked and golden brown.
4. When done, transfer fish patties to a plate lined with paper towels and let them rest until cooled.
5. Meanwhile, prepare the sauce and for this, place all the ingredients for the dip in a blender and pulse for 1 minute until smooth and creamy.
6. Place cooled fish cakes in batches in the meal prep glass containers and store in the refrigerator for up to 5 days or freeze for up to 3 months.
7. When ready to serve, microwave the fish cakes in their glass container for 1 to 2 minutes or until hot.

NUTRITION

- Calories: 69
- Fat: 6.5g
- Protein: 1.1g

- Net Carbs: 0.6g
- Fiber: 2.1g

PREPARATION: 15 MIN

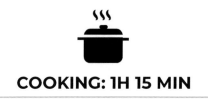

COOKING: 1H 15 MIN

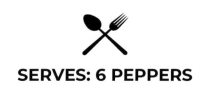

SERVES: 6 PEPPERS

LASAGNA STUFFED PEPPERS

INGREDIENTS

- 6 Large bell pepper, destemmed, cored
- 1 1/2 pound Ground beef, pastured
- 2 tablespoons Minced garlic
- ¾ teaspoon Sea salt
- ½ teaspoon Ground black pepper
- 2 cups Marinara sauce, organic
- 1 tablespoon Italian seasoning
- 1 cup Ricotta cheese, full-fat
- 1 cup Mozzarella cheese, full-fat, shredded

DIRECTIONS

1. Prepare the meat sauce and place a skillet pan over medium-high heat, grease with oil, and then add garlic and cook for 30 seconds until it is fragrant.
2. Then add beef, stir well, cook for 10 minutes until nicely browned, season with salt, black pepper and marinara sauce, stir well and simmer the sauce for 10 minutes.
3. Meanwhile, set an oven to 375 degrees F and let preheat.
4. When meat sauce is cooked, remove the pan from the oven and let cool for 5 minutes.
5. In the meantime, prepare the peppers and cut off the tops, then scoop the inside seeds and ribs and slice slightly from the bottoms, making no holes, so that peppers can stand upright.
6. Assemble the peppers and spoon 2 tablespoons of prepared meat sauce in the bottom of peppers, then evenly top with ricotta cheese and mozzarella cheese, and add two more layers in the same manner with mozzarella cheese on the top.
7. Take a baking sheet, line it with aluminum foil, place the stuffed peppers on it, and then tent with aluminum foil.
8. Place the baking sheet into the oven, bake for 30 minutes, remove the aluminum foil and continue baking for 10 minutes or until cheese melts and slightly browned.
9. Cool the stuffed pepper at room temperature, then wrap each pepper with aluminum foil and store in the freezer for about 2 to 3 minutes.
10. When ready to serve, reheat the peppers into the oven at 350 degrees F for 5 minutes or until hot.

NUTRITION

- Calories: 412
- Fat: 27g
- Protein: 30g
- Net Carbs: 8g
- Fiber: 2g

PREPARATION: 10 MIN

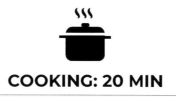

COOKING: 20 MIN

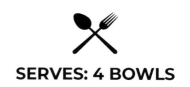

SERVES: 4 BOWLS

KOREAN GROUND BEEF BOWL

INGREDIENTS

- For Cauliflower Rice:
- 1 pound Cauliflower, riced
- 1/2 teaspoon Sea salt
- 1/8 teaspoon Ground black pepper
- 1 tablespoon Avocado oil
- For the Beef:
- 1 pound Beef, grass-fed
- 1/2 teaspoon Sea salt
- 2 tablespoons Minced garlic
- 1/4 cup Coconut aminos
- 1/4 teaspoon Ground ginger
- 1/4 teaspoon Crushed red pepper flakes
- 1 tablespoon Avocado oil
- 2 teaspoons Sesame oil
- 1/4 cup Beef broth, grass-fed
- For the Garnish:
- 1/4 cup Sliced Green onions
- 1 teaspoon Sesame seeds

DIRECTIONS

1. Prepare cauliflower rice and for this, take a large skillet pan, place it over medium-high heat, add oil and when hot, add cauliflower rice, season with salt and black pepper and cook for 5 minutes or until thoroughly cooked.
2. Then remove the pan from the heat, transfer to a bowl, and set aside until required.
3. Prepare the sauce, and for this, whisk together ginger, coconut aminos, red pepper flakes, sesame oil, and beef broth until combined, and set aside until required.
4. Return skillet pan over medium-high heat, add avocado oil and when hot, add beef, season with salt and cook for 10 minutes or light brown.
5. Make the well in the pan, add garlic to it, and cook for 1 minute or until sauté, then mix it into the beef and pour it in the prepared sauce.
6. Stir well and let beef simmer for 4 minutes or until sauce is thickened and not much liquid is left in the pan.
7. Remove pan from the heat and let beef cool completely.
8. Portion out the beef and cauliflower into four glass meal prep containers, garnish with green onion and sesame seeds, then cover with lid and store in the refrigerator for up to 5 days or freeze up to 2 months.
9. When ready to serve, reheat the beef and cauliflower in its glass container in the microwave for 1 to 2 minutes or until hot.

NUTRITION

- Calories: 513
- Fat: 36g
- Protein: 35g

- Net Carbs: 9g
- Fiber: 3g

PREPARATION: 15 MIN

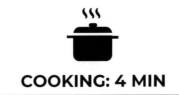
COOKING: 4 MIN

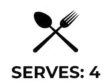
SERVES: 4

SALMON SKEWERS WRAPPED WITH PROSCIUTTO

INGREDIENTS

- ¼ cup basil
- 1 pound salmon
- 1 pinch of black pepper
- 4 ounces prosciutto
- 1 tbsp. olive oil
- 8 skewers

DIRECTIONS

1. Start by soaking the skewers in a bowl of water.
2. Cut the salmon fillets lengthwise. Thread the salmon using skewers.
3. Coat the skewers in pepper and basil. Wrap the slices of prosciutto around the salmon.
4. Warm-up oil in a grill pan. Grill the skewers within four minutes. Serve.

NUTRITION

- Calories: 670.5
- Protein: 27.2g
- Carbs: 1.2g
- Fat: 61.6g
- Fiber: 0.3g

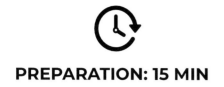
PREPARATION: 15 MIN

COOKING: 40 MIN

SERVES: 4

BUFFALO DRUMSTICKS AND CHILI AIOLI

INGREDIENTS

- For the chili aioli:
- ½ cup mayonnaise
- 1 tbsp. smoked paprika powder
- 1 garlic clove
- For the chicken:
- 2 pounds chicken drumsticks
- 2 tbsps. Of each:
- White wine vinegar
- Olive oil
- One tbsp. tomato paste
- 1 tsp. of each:
- Salt
- Paprika powder
- Tabasco

DIRECTIONS

1. Warm-up oven to 200 degrees.
2. Combine the listed marinade fixing. Marinate the chicken drumsticks within ten minutes.
3. Arrange the chicken drumsticks in the tray. Bake within forty minutes.
4. Combine the listed items for the chili aioli in a bowl. Serve.

NUTRITION

- Calories: 567.8
- Protein: 41.3g
- Carbs: 2.2g
- Fat: 43.2g
- Fiber: 1.1g

PREPARATION: 15 MIN

COOKING: 8H 15 MIN

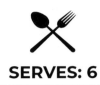
SERVES: 6

SLOW COOKED ROASTED PORK AND CREAMY GRAVY

INGREDIENTS

- For the creamy gravy:
- 2 cups whipping cream
- Roast juice
- For the pork:
- 2 pounds pork roast
- 1/2 tbsp. Salt
- 1 bay leaf
- 5 black peppercorns
- 3 cups of water
- 2 tsp. thyme
- 2 garlic cloves
- 2 ounces ginger
- 1 tbsp. of each:
- Paprika powder
- Olive oil
- 1/3 tsp. black pepper

DIRECTIONS

1. Warm-up your oven to 100 degrees.
2. Add the meat, salt, water to a baking dish. Put peppercorns, thyme, and bay leaf. Put in the oven within eight hours. Remove. Reserve the juices. Adjust to 200 degrees.
3. Put ginger, garlic, pepper, herbs, and oil. Rub the herb mixture on the meat. Roast the pork within fifteen minutes.
4. Slice the roasted meat. Strain the meat juices in a bowl. Boil for reducing it by half.
5. Add the cream. Simmer within twenty minutes. Serve with creamy gravy.

NUTRITION

- Calories: 586.9
- Protein: 27.9g
- Carbs: 2.6g
- Fat: 50.3g
- Fiber: 1.5g

PREPARATION: 15 MIN **COOKING: 1 HOUR** **SERVES: 4**

BACON-WRAPPED MEATLOAF

INGREDIENTS

- For the meatloaf:
- 2 tbsps. butter
- 1 onion
- 2 pounds beef
- 1/2 cup whipping cream
- 2 ounces cheese
- 1 large egg
- 1 tbsp. oregano
- 1 tsp. Salt
- 1/2 tsp. black pepper
- 7 ounces bacon
- For the gravy:
- 1& 1/2 cup whipping cream
- 1/2 tbsp. tamari soy sauce

DIRECTIONS

1. Warm-up your oven to 200 degrees Celsius.
2. Dissolve the butter in a pan. Add the onion. Cook within four minutes. Keep aside.
3. Combine onion, ground meat, and the remaining fixing except for the bacon in a large bowl.
4. Make a firm loaf. Use bacon strips for wrapping the loaf.
5. Bake the meatloaf for forty-five minutes.
6. Put the juices from the baking dish and cream, then boil. Simmer within ten minutes. Add the soy sauce. Slice and serve with gravy.

NUTRITION

- Calories: 1020.3
- Protein: 46.7g
- Carbs: 5.6g
- Fat: 88.9g
- Fiber: 1.2g

PREPARATION: 15 MIN

COOKING: 4 MIN

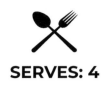
SERVES: 4

LAMB CHOPS AND HERB BUTTER

INGREDIENTS

- 8 lamb chops
- 1 tbsp. Each:
- Olive oil
- Butter
- Pepper
- Salt
- For the herb butter:
- 5 ounces butter
- 1 clove garlic
- 1/2 tbsp. garlic powder
- 4 tbsps. parsley
- 1 tsp. lemon juice
- 1/3 tsp. Salt

DIRECTIONS

1. Season the lamb chops with pepper and salt.
2. Warm-up olive oil and butter in an iron skillet. Add the lamb chops. Fry within four minutes.
3. Mix all the listed items for the herb butter in a bowl. Cool.
4. Serve with herb butter.

NUTRITION

- Calories: 722.3
- Protein: 42.3g
- Carbs: 0.4g
- Fat: 61.5g
- Fiber: 0.4g

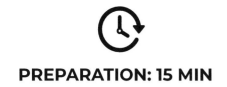

PREPARATION: 15 MIN

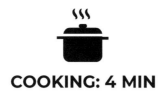

COOKING: 4 MIN

SERVES: 6

CRISPY CUBAN PORK ROAST

INGREDIENTS

- 5 pounds pork shoulder
- 4 tsp. Salt
- 2 tsp. cumin
- 1 tsp. black pepper
- 2 tbsps. oregano
- 1 red onion
- 4 garlic cloves
- Orange juice
- Lemons juice
- One-fourth cup of olive oil

DIRECTIONS

1. Rub the pork shoulder with salt in a bowl. Mix all the remaining items of the marinade in a blender.
2. Marinate the meat within eight hours. Cook within forty minutes. Warm-up your oven to 200 degrees. Roast the pork within thirty minutes.
3. Remove the meat juice. Simmer within twenty minutes. Shred the meat.
4. Pour the meat juice. Serve.

NUTRITION

- Calories: 910.3
- Protein: 58.3g
- Carbs: 5.3g
- Fat: 69.6g
- Fiber: 2.2g

PREPARATION: 15 MIN

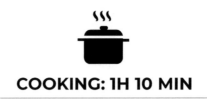
COOKING: 1H 10 MIN

SERVES: 4

KETO BARBECUED RIBS

INGREDIENTS

- 1/4 cup Dijon mustard
- 2 tbsps. Of each:
- Cider vinegar
- Butter
- Salt
- 3 pounds of spare ribs
- 4 tbsps. paprika powder
- 1/2 tbsp. chili powder
- 1&1/2 tbsp. garlic powder
- 2 tsp. of each:
- Onion powder
- Cumin
- Two & 1/2 tbsp. black pepper

DIRECTIONS

1. Warm-up a grill for thirty minutes.
2. Mix vinegar and Dijon mustard in a bowl put the ribs, and coat.
3. Mix all the listed spices. Rub the mix all over the ribs. Put aside. Put ribs on an aluminum foil. Add some butter over the ribs. Wrap with foil. Grill within one hour. Remove and slice.
4. Put the reserved spice mix. Grill again within ten minutes. Serve.

NUTRITION

- Calories: 980.3
- Protein: 54.3g
- Carbs: 5.8g
- Fat: 80.2g

PREPARATION: 15 MIN

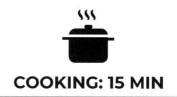

COOKING: 15 MIN

SERVES: 4

SKINNY BANG BANG ZUCCHINI NOODLES

INGREDIENTS

- For the noodles:
- 4 medium zucchini spiraled
- 1 tbsp. olive oil
- For the sauce:
- 0.25 cup + 2 tablespoons Plain Greek Yogurt
- 0.25 cup + 2 tablespoons Mayo
- 0.25 cup + 2 tablespoons Thai Sweet Chili Sauce
- 1.5 teaspoons Honey
- 1.5 teaspoons Sriracha
- 2 teaspoons Lime Juice

DIRECTIONS

1. If you are using any meats for this dish, such as chicken or shrimp, cook them first, then set aside.
2. Pour the oil into a large-sized skillet at medium temperature.
3. After the oil heats through, stir in the spiraled zucchini noodles.
4. Cook the "noodles" until tender yet still crispy.
5. Remove from the heat, drain, and set at rest for at least 10 minutes.
6. Combine sauce items into a large-sized, both until perfectly smooth.
7. Give it a taste & adjust as needed.
8. Divide into 4 small containers. Mix your noodles with any meats you cooked and add them to meal prep containers.
9. When you're ready to eat it, heat the noodles, drain any excess water, and mix in the sauce.

NUTRITION

- Net carbs: 18g
- Fiber: 0g
- Fat: 1g
- Protein: 9g
- Calories: 161g

PREPARATION: 15 MIN

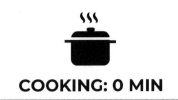

COOKING: 0 MIN

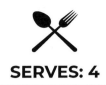

SERVES: 4

KETO CAESAR SALAD

INGREDIENTS

- 1.5 cups Mayonnaise
- 3 tablespoons Apple Cider Vinegar/ACV
- 1 teaspoon Dijon Mustard
- 4 Anchovy Fillet
- 24 Romaine Heart Leaves
- 4 ounces, Pork Rinds, chopped
- Parmesan (for garnish)

DIRECTIONS

1. Place the mayo with ACV, mustard, and anchovies into a blender and process until smooth and dressing.
2. Prepare romaine leaves and pour out, dressing across them evenly.
3. Top with pork rinds and enjoy.

NUTRITION

- Net carbs: 4g
- Fiber: 3g
- Fat: 86g
- Protein: 47g
- Calories: 993kcal

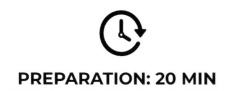 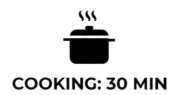

PREPARATION: 20 MIN   **COOKING: 30 MIN**   **SERVES: 6**

KETO BUFFALO CHICKEN EMPANADAS

INGREDIENTS

- For the empanada dough:
- 1 ½ cups of mozzarella cheese
- 3 oz. of cream cheese
- 1 whisked egg
- 2 cups of almond flour
- For the buffalo chicken filling:
- 2 cups of cooked shredded chicken
- 2 tablespoons Butter, melted
- 0.33 cup Hot Sauce

DIRECTIONS

1. Bring the oven to a temperature of 425-degrees.
2. Put the cheese & cream cheese into a microwave-safe dish. Microwave at 1-minute intervals until completely combined.
3. Stir the flour and egg into the dish until it is well-combined. Add any additional flour for consistency—until it stops sticking to your fingers.
4. With another medium-sized bowl, combine the chicken with sauce and set aside.
5. Cover a flat surface with plastic wrap or parchment paper and sprinkle with almond flour.
6. Spray a rolling pin to avoid sticking and use it to press the dough flat.
7. Make circle shapes out of this dough with a lid, a cup, or a cookie-cutter. For the excess dough, roll back up and repeat the process.
8. Portion out spoonful of filling into these dough circles but keep them only on one half.
9. Fold the other half over to close up into half-moon shapes. Press on the edges to seal them.
10. Lay on a lightly greased cooking sheet and bake for around 9 minutes until perfectly brown.

NUTRITION

- Net carbs: 20g
- Fiber: 0g
- Fat: 96g

- Protein: 74g
- Calories: 1217kcal

PREPARATION: 15 MIN

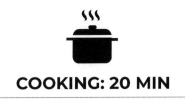
COOKING: 20 MIN

SERVES: 3

PEPPERONI AND CHEDDAR STROMBOLI

INGREDIENTS

- 1.25 cups Mozzarella Cheese
- 0.25 cup Almond Flour
- 3 tablespoons Coconut Flour
- 1 teaspoon Italian Seasoning
- 1 large-sized Egg, whisked
- 6 ounces Deli Ham, sliced
- 2 ounces Pepperoni, sliced
- 4 ounces Cheddar Cheese, sliced
- 1 tablespoon Butter, melted
- 6 cups Salad Greens

DIRECTIONS

1. First, bring the oven to a temperature of 400 degrees and prepare a baking tray with some parchment paper.
2. Use the microwave to melt the mozzarella until it can be stirred.
3. Mix flours & Italian seasoning in a separate small-sized bowl.
4. Dump in the melty cheese and stir together with pepper and salt to taste.
5. Stir in the egg and process the dough with your hands. Pour it onto that prepared baking tray.
6. Roll out the dough w/ your hands or a pin. Cut slits that mark out 4 equal rectangles.
7. Put the ham and cheese onto the dough, then brush with butter and close up, putting the seal end down.
8. Bake for around 17 minutes until well-browned. Slice up and serve.

NUTRITION

- Net carbs: 20g
- Fiber: 0g
- Fat: 13g
- Protein: 11g
- Calories: 240kcal

PREPARATION: 15 MIN

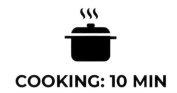

COOKING: 10 MIN

SERVES: 4

TUNA CASSEROLE

INGREDIENTS

- 16 Ounces Tuna in oil, drained
- 2 tablespoons Butter
- 1/2 teaspoon Salt
- 1 teaspoon Black pepper
- 1 teaspoon Chili powder
- 6 stalks Celery
- 1 Green bell pepper
- 1 Yellow onion
- 4 ounces Parmesan cheese, grated
- 1 cup Mayonnaise

DIRECTIONS

1. Heat the oven to 400°
2. Chop the onion, bell pepper, and celery very fine and fry in the melted butter for five minutes.
3. Stir together with the chili powder, parmesan cheese, tuna, and mayonnaise.
4. Use lard to grease an eight by eight-inch or nine by a nine-inch baking pan.
5. Add the tuna mixture into the fried vegetables and spoon the mix into the baking pan.
6. Bake it for twenty minutes.

NUTRITION

- Calories: 953
- Net Carbs: 5g
- Fat: 83g

- Protein: 43g

PREPARATION: 15 MIN

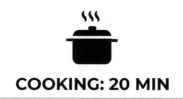
COOKING: 20 MIN

SERVES: 4

BRUSSELS SPROUT AND HAMBURGER GRATIN

INGREDIENTS

- 1 pound Ground beef
- 8 ounces Bacon, diced small
- 15 ounces Brussels sprouts, cut in half
- 1 teaspoon Salt
- 1 teaspoon Black pepper
- ½ teaspoon Thyme
- 1 cup Cheddar cheese, shredded
- 1 tablespoon Italian seasoning
- 4 tablespoons Sour cream
- 2 tablespoons Butter

DIRECTIONS

1. Heat the oven to 425°.
2. Fry bacon and Brussels sprouts in butter for five minutes.
3. Stir in the sour cream and pour this mix into a greased eight by an eight-inch baking pan.
4. Cook the ground beef and season with the salt and pepper, then add this mix to the baking pan.
5. Top with the herbs and the shredded cheese. Bake for twenty minutes.

NUTRITION

- Calories: 770kcal
- Net carbs: 8g
- Fat: 62g
- Protein: 42g

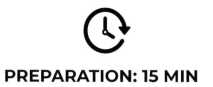

PREPARATION: 15 MIN

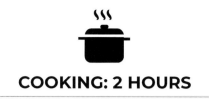

COOKING: 2 HOURS

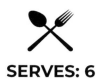

SERVES: 6

BACON APPETIZERS

INGREDIENTS

- 1 pack Keto crackers
- ¾ cup Parmesan cheese, grated
- 1 lb. bacon, sliced thinly

DIRECTIONS

1. Preheat your oven to 250 degrees F.
2. Arrange the crackers on a baking sheet.
3. Sprinkle cheese on top of each cracker.
4. Wrap each cracker with the bacon.
5. Bake in the oven for 2 hours.

NUTRITION

- Calories: 440
- Total Fat: 33.4g
- Saturated Fat: 11g
- Cholesterol: 86mg
- Sodium: 1813mg
- Total Carbohydrate: 3.7g
- Dietary Fiber: 0.1g
- Total Sugars: 0.1g
- Protein: 29.4g
- Potassium: 432mg

11. DINNER

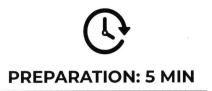
PREPARATION: 5 MIN

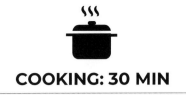
COOKING: 30 MIN

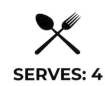
SERVES: 4

ANGRY ALFREDO FROM OLIVE GARDEN

INGREDIENTS

- For the Sauce:
- ½ cup of parmesan cheese, freshly grated
- 4 oz. of butter
- ½ tsp. garlic powder
- 1 cup of heavy cream
- ¼ tsp. red pepper chili flakes
- For the Chicken:
- Salt & pepper
- 8 oz. breast of chicken
- 1 tbsp. olive oil
- For the Topping:
- ½ cup of mozzarella cheese

DIRECTIONS

1. Make the sauce. Warm a saucepan using the med-high heat setting to melt the butter. Be careful that the butter does not turn brown. Add the heavy cream, and wait till bubbles are formed. When bubbles begin to appear, add the cheese. Stir the ingredients frequently to ensure the sauce thickens to create a smooth consistency. Adjust the temperature to simmer on the stovetop. Add in the garlic powder and crushed pepper to the sauce.
2. Prepare the chicken. Use salt and pepper and season the chicken. You need a medium-sized skillet; a cast-iron skillet is preferred. Heat it over the med-high flame to warm two tablespoons of olive oil.
3. Cook the chicken for around five minutes or for a maximum of seven minutes. Once the edges turn white, this is the right time to flip the chicken breast. Keep cooking until the chicken is thoroughly cooked or for another five minutes or up to seven minutes.
4. Finish it. Set the oven to broil and preheat it. By now, the chicken is done. Allow it to rest and cool for some time (five minutes).
5. Dice the chicken into small chunks, so they are bite-sized. Mix the chicken with the Alfredo sauce. Place this into the casserole dish of one-quart size. Use mozzarella cheese as a topping, and place the casserole dish below the broiler. Wait till the cheese turns brown. When the cheese begins to turn brown, transfer it from the oven.

Note: The appetizer is served with sliced baguette bread—usually. If you want to keep it keto-friendly, use a low-carb bread or low-carb crackers. This also helps in checking the carbohydrates you consume with this appetizer accompaniment.

NUTRITION

- Calories: 596
- Carbs: 2g
- Protein: 21g
- Fat: 56g
- Fiber: 32g

PREPARATION: 30 MIN

COOKING: 3H 40 MIN

SERVES: 9

BEEF BARBACOA AT CHIPOTLE-SLOW-COOKED

INGREDIENTS

- 2 medium chipotle chills in adobo + 4 tsp. sauce
- 3 ½ cups beef/chicken broth
- 2 tbsp. apple cider vinegar
- 5 minced garlic cloves
- 2 tbsp. lime juice
- 2 tsp. cumin
- 2 whole bay leaves
- 1 tbsp. dried oregano
- 1 tsp. black pepper
- 2 tsp. sea salt
- Optional Ingredient: ½ tsp. ground cloves
- 3 lb. chuck roast/Beef brisket

DIRECTIONS

1. Trim the beef into two-inch chunks.
2. Combine the chipotle chills with the sauce, broth, lime juice, garlic, vinegar, oregano, sea salt, cumin, ground cloves, and black pepper into a blender (all but the beef and bay leaves). Puree until smooth.
3. Toss the chunks of beef, the pureed mixture from the blender, and the whole bay leaves into the slow cooker.
4. Cook for four to six hours on high or eight to ten hours on low until the beef is tender and falling apart.
5. Trash the bay leaves, shred the meat using two forks, and stir into the juices.
6. Cover and allow the flavors mix for five to ten minutes. Use a slotted spoon to serve.

NUTRITION

- Calories: 242
- Protein: 32g
- Carbs: 2g
- Fat: 11g
- Fiber: 1g

PREPARATION: 10 MIN

COOKING: 15 MIN

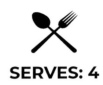
SERVES: 4

BEEF & BROCCOLI FROM PF CHANG'S

INGREDIENTS

- 1 lb. of beef–ex. sirloin, skirt steak, or flank steak
- 2-3 cloves garlic
- 1-2 heads broccoli, broken into florets (or pre-cut bagged)
- 2 pieces of ginger
- Ghee or olive oil
- Optional to Garnish:
- Sesame seeds
- Chopped scallions
- The Marinade:
- 1 tbsp. + 2.5 tsp. sesame oil
- 1 tbsp. Red Boat Fish Sauce
- 4 tbsp. coconut aminos - divided
- ¼ tsp. - baking soda
- ½ tsp. sea salt
- 3 minced garlic cloves
- 1 tsp. - ginger
- ½ tsp. of black pepper - divided
- Optional: ¼ tsp. crushed red pepper

DIRECTIONS

1. Combine the ingredients for the marinade and sauce (in two separate bowls) and set aside.
2. The Marinade: Two tablespoons of coconut aminos, ½ teaspoon of salt, one tablespoon of sesame oil, and ¼ teaspoon of baking soda.
3. The Sauce: Mix the stir fry sauce by combining two tablespoons coconut aminos, one tablespoon fish sauce, two teaspoons sesame oil, and pepper.
4. Slice the beef into ¼-inch thin slices and place in a pan with the marinade for at least 15 minutes.
5. Chop the broccoli (or take it out the bag if using pre-cut). Put it in a safe microwave bowl with two tablespoons of water and cover. Microwave for two to three minutes until it is tender but still has a crunch. Place it to the side for now.
6. Warm a skillet or wok using the med-high temperature setting along with one tablespoon olive oil or ghee. Mince and add the garlic, ginger, and salt. Sauté them for about 15 seconds.
7. Crank the temperature setting to high and add the marinated beef. Be sure to evenly distribute it and cook for around two minutes (without moving it about too much) until the edges are dark—then flip and repeat.
8. Final Step: Add the sauce and stir-fry for about one minute. Mix in the broccoli.
9. Toss it further for another ½ minute and toss to serve.

Note: This recipe calls for coconut aminos, but you may substitute it with a gluten-free soy sauce or Tamari. However, you will need to use half the amount to achieve a more robust, saltier flavor. Have you ever used Red Boat Fish Sauce before? It is a Vietnamese fish sauce that pro chefs often use to create that elusive "fifth flavor-umami." It is made using black anchovy and sea salt with no added msg or preservatives. Each tablespoon of the sauce has 4grams of protein, 15 calories, and -0- carbs and sugar. It is gluten-free and keto-friendly. Remember, this is the secret to the recipe: For this Keto Beef and Broccoli to be on point, you need to marinate the slices of beef for at least 15 minutes.

NUTRITION

- Calories: 255
- Protein: 28.2g
- Carbs: 9.2g
- Fat: 12.4g
- Fiber: 2.4g

PREPARATION: 10 MIN

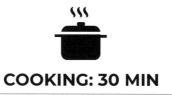
COOKING: 30 MIN

SERVES: 4

CHICKEN SALAD FROM CHICKEN SALAD CHICK

INGREDIENTS

- 32 oz. of low-sodium chicken stock
- ½ tsp. salt
- ½ cup of mayonnaise
- 1 ½ lb. chicken tenders
- 2 tbsp. celery–finely minced
- ½ tsp. ground black pepper
- 2 tsp. dry ranch salad dressing mix

DIRECTIONS

1. Poach the chicken in the chicken stock. Use an oversized pot to prepare the chicken stock and chicken tenders. Poach them for 15 minutes. You can extend by another five minutes to cook or until the chicken is thoroughly done—not pinkish.
2. The next step is to shred the chicken. You can use one of two methods for this. Choose a paddle attachment and shred with the stand mixer. The chicken tenders can also be shredded with two forks.
3. Take a bowl that is of medium-size. To this, add mayonnaise, dry Ranch dressing mix, celery, black pepper, and salt. Stir these well, and combine thoroughly. They should be blended well.
4. To this mixture, add the shredded chicken. Again mix thoroughly. You need to store this chicken salad for future use in an air-tight container.
5. If you want better results, you need to prepare the chicken salad a few hours before eating or serving it.
6. You can use this to serve with a sandwich or with bread lettuce. You can also serve it with any dish of your choice.
7. If you want to bring in more variety, add a tablespoon or two tablespoons of green bell pepper. You can place this in any container that does not let air escape. You can store in air-tight containers for a maximum of four days.
8. If you want to make this recipe gluten-free, you need to check the ingredients' labels. Some store-bought chicken stock contains gluten. Avoid them if you are on a gluten-free diet.

NUTRITION

- Calories: 430
- Carbs: 5g
- Protein: 41g
- Fat: 27g
- Fiber: 1g

PREPARATION: 5 MIN

COOKING: 20 MIN

SERVES: 4

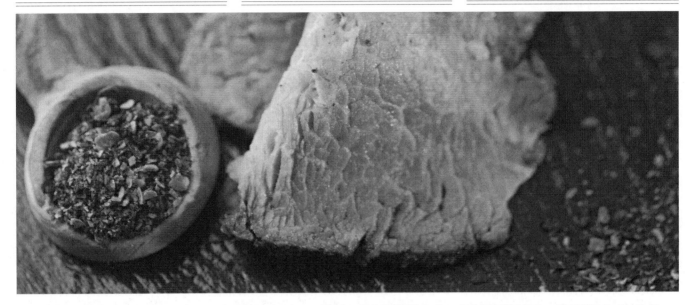

CHIPOTLE GRILL GLUTEN-FREE STEAK BOWL

INGREDIENTS

- 16 oz. skirt steak
- Black pepper & salt
- 1 homemade guacamole recipe
- 1 cup sour cream
- 1 handful fresh cilantro
- 4 oz. pepper jack cheese
- 1 splash Chipotle Tabasco Sauce

DIRECTIONS

1. Prepare the steak with a dusting of pepper and salt. Warm a cast-iron skillet using the high-temperature setting. Once hot, add the steak to cook for three to four minutes per side. Let it rest on a plate while you prepare the guacamole.
2. Prepare the guacamole according to the below recipe.
3. Slice the steak against the grain into thin, bite-sized strips (4 portions).
4. Shred the pepper jack cheese using a cheese grater and sprinkle it over the steak.
5. Add about ¼ cup of guacamole to each portion, followed by ¼ cup of sour cream.
6. Splash each portion with sauce and fresh cilantro to serve.

NUTRITION

- Calories: 620
- Protein: 33g
- Net Carbs: 5.5g
- Fat: 50g

PREPARATION: 5 MIN

COOKING: 10 MIN

SERVES: 1

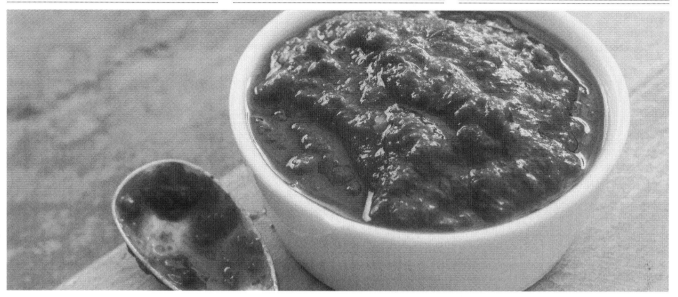

CHIPOTLE GUACAMOLE SAUCE

INGREDIENTS

- 2 ripe avocados
- 1 lime
- ¼ cup red onion
- 6 grape tomatoes
- 1 garlic clove
- 1 tbsp. olive oil
- ⅛ tsp. black pepper
- ¼ tsp. salt
- Fresh cilantro
- Optional: ⅛ tsp. crushed red pepper

DIRECTIONS

1. Do the prep. Juice the lime. Slice, remove the pit, and mash the avocados in a mixing container.
2. Dice the tomatoes and red onions. Add them to the avocado.
3. Mince the garlic clove and add the oil to combine.
4. Stir in the cilantro with the salt, pepper, crushed red pepper, and lime juice.
5. Thoroughly mix and serve with a steak bowl and a portion of pork rinds or low-carb crackers.

NUTRITION

- Calories: 155
- Protein: 2g
- Carbs: 2g

- Fat: 14g

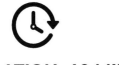
PREPARATION: 40 MIN

COOKING: 3H 30 MIN

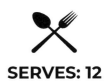
SERVES: 12

CHIPOTLE PORK CARNITAS FROM CHIPOTLE

INGREDIENTS

- 2 tbsp. of sunflower oil
- 4 lb. pork roast
- 1 tsp. salt
- 1 cup of water
- 1 tsp. thyme
- 2 tsp. juniper berries
- ½ tsp. ground black pepper

DIRECTIONS

1. Set the temperature of your oven to 300 degrees Fahrenheit. This is to preheat the oven.
2. In the Dutch oven, add sunflower oil in medium flame. Use salt to season the roast. Once the oil is heated, sauté the roast on all sides. This will take three minutes per side.
3. You will brown the roast a bit when you sauté this way. You need to add bay leaves, juniper berries, water, thyme, and ground black pepper to the Dutch oven.
4. Close the pan with the lid. Cook this in the oven for three to four hours. In the pot, you need to keep turning the roast frequently. Only then, the flavors will get into the roast, and it will incorporate the taste.
5. Take off the roast from the oven. Rest this for 20 minutes. Use two forks to pull the meat out of the pot.
6. Slow Cooker Directions: To a large skillet, add the sunflower oil. You can also add it to the Dutch oven and warm it using medium heat. When the oil gets hot, sauté the roast.
7. Place the meat into the slow cooker and add water, ground black pepper, thyme, bay leaves, and juniper berries.
8. Cover the cooker with a lid. Cook the meat for three to four hours using medium heat throughout the process. While cooking, turn the roast once in an hour or once in 45 minutes or so. While you keep turning the roast less frequently, in this manner, you can ensure that the flavors get into the roast with ease.
9. If you want to use a pressure cooker for this recipe, it is not recommended. Only a slow cooker will ensure that the meat gets the perfect flavor. A fast cooking process using a pressure cooker will not give it a delicious flavor.
10. When you are choosing the pork, choose the cut that has marbling. Do not worry about the fat. You can always trim it.
11. If you do not prefer juniper berries, you can omit them. But the flavor would be altered when omitting juniper berries.

Note: For making the recipe keto-friendly, you can bring in avocado oil as a substitute to the sunflower oil.

NUTRITION

- Calories: 223
- Carbs: 0g
- Protein: 33g
- Fat: 8g
- Fiber: 0g

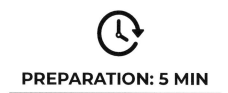

PREPARATION: 5 MIN

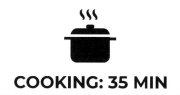

COOKING: 35 MIN

SERVES: 4

CRAWFISH ETOUFFEE FROM MAGNOLIA BAR AND GRILL

INGREDIENTS

- ½ cup of butter
- 1 tsp. flour
- ¼ tsp. cayenne pepper
- 1 lb. cleaned crawfish tails
- 2 thin slices of lemon
- 1 tbsp. green onion
- 1 tbsp. tomato paste
- 1 medium onion
- 1 tsp. salt
- 1 tbsp. parsley

DIRECTIONS

1. To make the Etouffee, make use of a saucepan with a lid that tightly fits.
2. Use salt and pepper to season the crawfish tails. Keep the seasoned crawfish tails to the side.
3. Melt the butter in the pan. Finely chop and toss in the onions once the butter melts. Sauté the chopped onions over medium flame. Turn off the burner. Add the flour to the cooked onions. Stir and thoroughly combine them.
4. Then add ¾ cup of water—followed by lemon and tomato paste. Simmer and cook slowly for another 20 minutes. Keep adding water slowly, and less frequently.
5. When the sauce is cooked after 20 minutes, add the seasoned crawfish tails. Cover the saucepan with the lid. Cook again for eight more minutes.
6. Add salt and pepper, and check the seasoning for taste.
7. Now, add the parsley and green onion. Cook it for two more minutes. This goes well with steamed rice. Serve it hot.

Note: The recipe goes perfectly with white and brown rice. You can also serve it with spinach pasta, grits, and chopped and cooked cauliflower.

NUTRITION

- Calories: 237
- Protein: 3g
- Carbs: 5g
- Fat: 23g
- Fiber: 0g

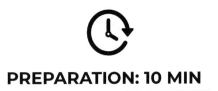
PREPARATION: 10 MIN

COOKING: 50 MIN

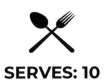
SERVES: 10

HASH-BROWN CASSEROLE FROM CRACKER BARREL

INGREDIENTS

- 1 pint of sour cream
- ½ cup margarine/butter, melted
- 1 lb. frozen hash-browns
- 1 10.25 oz. can cream of chicken soup
- ½ cup of onion
- 1 tsp. salt
- 2 cups of grated cheddar cheese
- ¼ tsp. pepper

DIRECTIONS

1. Preheat the oven. Set the temperature at 350 degrees Fahrenheit. Use an 11 x 14 baking dish. Spray it with cooking spray.
2. Peel and chop the onion. Mix the margarine or butter, sour cream, frozen hash-browns, cream of chicken soup, onions, salt, pepper, and cheddar cheese. Combine them well, and transfer to the baking pan you have prepared.
3. Set a timer to bake for 45 minutes. You need to check if the top has become browned or done cooking at this stage.

Note: This comes handy when you have many people to feed or as a suitable recipe for brunch.

NUTRITION

- Calories: 488.4
- Carbs: 30.1g
- Protein: 10.3g
- Fat: 37.8g
- Fiber: 2g

PREPARATION: 5 MIN

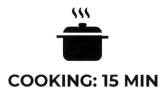
COOKING: 15 MIN

SERVES: 6

SOUTHWESTERN EGG ROLLS FROM CHILIES

INGREDIENTS

- Smoked Chicken Ingredients:
- 1 tsp. of olive/vegetable oil
- 8 oz. chicken breast
- Egg Roll Filling:
- ¼ cup of green onions, minced
- ¼ cup of red bell peppers, minced
- 1 tbsp. of olive oil (Alternatively, vegetable oil can be used)
- ½ cup of frozen corn
- ¼ cup of frozen spinach, drained & thawed
- ½ cup of black beans from a can, drained & rinsed
- 1 tsp. of taco seasoning
- 8 seven-inch flour tortillas
- 2 tsp. pickled jalapeno peppers, chopped
- ¾ cup of shredded jack cheese
- Avocado Ranch Ingredients:
- ½ cup of milk
- ½ cup of mayonnaise
- ¼ cup of mashed fresh avocados (approximately half an avocado)
- 1 package Ranch dressing mix
- Toppings:
- 1 tbsp. chopped onions
- 2 tbsp. chopped tomatoes

DIRECTIONS

1. Cook the breast of chicken. Start with seasoning the chicken with salt and pepper. Use a brush and apply the olive oil or vegetable oil on the chicken breast. On a medium-hot grill, grill the chicken.
2. Cook the chicken five to seven minutes on one side. When done, flip and cook the other side for another five to seven minutes. Cut the chicken into small pieces. Set it aside while you carry on with the next step.
3. Prepare the Egg Roll Filling: Sauté the red pepper. It should become tender. To this, add pickled jalapenos, black beans, spinach, corn, and green onion. After adding these, add the taco seasoning. Heat the mixture thoroughly.
4. On the tortillas, place an equal amount of the filling. Then place an equal amount of chicken. Top them with cheese. Fold the ends, and roll the tortillas up. They should be rolled very tight to prevent the fillings from coming off. You can also use toothpicks to secure the tortillas from opening. Pin with these after folding.
5. Cook the egg rolls. Use a large pot and add about four inches of oil into the pot. Heat to reach a temperature of 350 degrees Fahrenheit. In the heated oil, deep fry the tortillas. They should turn golden brown. For this, it might take around seven to eight minutes. When they are golden brown, take off from the oil. Then keep them on a wire rack.
6. Prepare the Avocado Ranch Dressing. In a bowl mix, half a cup of mayonnaise, half a cup of buttermilk with the package of Ranch dressing mix. When thoroughly combined, add mashed avocado of a quarter cup to this mixture. In a blender, transfer this mixture. Blend in pulse option. The dipping sauce should become smooth, and when blended perfectly, stop pulsing.

NUTRITION

- Calories: 502
- Carbs: 21g
- Protein: 19g

- Fat: 28g
- Fiber: 3g

PREPARATION: 5 MIN

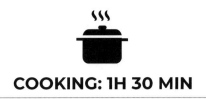
COOKING: 1H 30 MIN

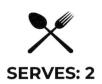
SERVES: 2

LAMB SHANKS

INGREDIENTS

- 1/4 cup Avocado oil
- 2.5 pounds Lamb shanks
- 1 tablespoon Minced garlic
- 1 Medium white onion, peeled and diced
- 2 Sticks of celery, diced
- 2 tablespoons Rosemary
- 1 teaspoon Salt
- 1/2 teaspoon Ground black pepper
- 1 cup Lamb or chicken broth
- 14 ounces Diced tomatoes

DIRECTIONS

1. Switch on the instant pot, add half of the oil, press the 'sauté/simmer' button, wait until the oil is hot and lamb shanks in a single layer and cook for 3 to 5 minutes per side or until browned.
2. Transfer lamb shanks to a plate, set aside, then add onion, celery, garlic, and rosemary into the instant pot and cook for 3 minutes.
3. Season with salt and black pepper, pour in the broth, mix well, then add tomatoes, return lamb shanks into the pot and toss until combined.
4. Press the 'keep warm' button, shut the instant pot with its lid in the sealed position, then press the 'manual' button, press '+/-' to set the cooking time to 50 minutes and cook at high-pressure setting; when the pressure builds in the pot, the cooking timer will start.
5. When the instant pot buzzes, press the 'keep warm' button, release pressure naturally for 10 minutes, then do a quick pressure release and open the lid.
6. Transfer lamb shanks to a dish, then press the 'sauté/simmer' button and simmer the sauce for 5 minutes or more until the sauce is reduced by half.
7. Ladle sauce over the lamb shanks and serve.

NUTRITION

- Calories: 410
- Fat: 35g
- Protein: 51g
- Net Carbs: 12g
- Fiber: 3g

PREPARATION: 10 MIN

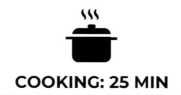

COOKING: 25 MIN

SERVES: 4

ZUPPA TOSCANA

INGREDIENTS

- 6 Slices of bacon, chopped
- 1 pound Ground Italian sausage
- 1 tablespoon Butter, unsalted
- 2 teaspoons Minced garlic
- ½ teaspoon Ground sage
- ¼ teaspoon Ground black pepper
- 2 ¾ cups Chicken broth
- ¾ cup Heavy whipping cream
- ¼ cup Parmesan cheese, shredded
- 1 pound Radishes, peeled, quartered
- 2 ounces Kale, de-stemmed, leaves chopped

DIRECTIONS

1. Switch on the instant pot, grease pot with oil, press the 'sauté/simmer' button, wait until the oil is hot, add sausage and cook for 5 minutes or until browned.
2. Transfer sausage to a plate, add bacon in the pot and cook for 4 minutes or until crispy.
3. Transfer bacon to a cutting board, let sit for 5 minutes and then chop it.
4. Add garlic in the instant pot, cook for 1 minute or until fragrant, then return sausage and bacon into the pot, add remaining ingredients except for cream, cheese, and kale and stir until mixed.
5. Press the 'keep warm' button, shut the instant pot with its lid in the sealed position, then press the 'manual' button, press '+/-' to set the cooking time to 10 minutes and cook at high-pressure setting; when the pressure builds in the pot, the cooking timer will start.
6. When the instant pot buzzes, press the 'keep warm' button, do a quick pressure release and open the lid.
7. Add remaining ingredients, stir well, press the 'sauté/simmer' button and simmer the soup for 5 minutes or until kale is tender.
8. Ladle soup into bowls and serve.

NUTRITION

- Calories: 316
- Fat: 25g
- Protein: 13g
- Net Carbs: 6g
- Fiber: 3g

PREPARATION: 10 MIN

COOKING: 7H 15 MIN

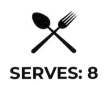
SERVES: 8

MEXICAN SHREDDED BEEF

INGREDIENTS

- 3 1/2 pounds Beef short ribs, grass-fed
- 2 tablespoons Minced garlic
- 2 teaspoons Ground turmeric
- 1 teaspoon Salt
- 1/2 teaspoon Ground black pepper
- 2 teaspoons Ground cumin
- 2 teaspoons Ground coriander
- 1 teaspoon Chipotle powder
- 1/2 cup Water
- 1 cup Cilantro stems, chopped

DIRECTIONS

1. Place salt in a small bowl, add black pepper, cumin, coriander, chipotle powder and stir until mixed.
2. Place ribs into the slow cooker, sprinkle well with the prepared spice mix and then top with minced garlic and cilantro stems.
3. Switch on the slow cooker, pour in water, then cover with the lid and cook for 6 to 7 hours over low heat setting or until tender.
4. Then pour the sauce into a small saucepan and cook for 10 to 15 minutes or until reduced by half.
5. Return the sauce into the slow cooker, pull apart the meat and toss until well mixed.
6. Portion out beef into eight glass meal prep containers, then cover with lid and store in the refrigerator for up to 5 days or freeze for up to 2 months.
7. When ready to serve, reheat the beef in its glass container in the microwave for 1 to 2 minutes or until hot.

NUTRITION

- Calories: 656
- Fat: 48.5g
- Protein: 50.2g

- Net Carbs: 1g
- Fiber: 0.4g

PREPARATION: 5 MIN

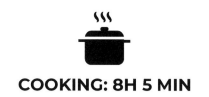

COOKING: 8H 5 MIN

SERVES: 4

BEEF STEW

INGREDIENTS

- 3 1/2 pounds Beef, grass-fed, diced
- 3 Stalks of celery, chopped
- 1 Leek, white part only
- 15 ounces Diced tomatoes
- ¾ cup Spinach leaves, fresh
- 3 Carrots, chopped into large rounds
- 1 tablespoon Chopped ginger
- ½ tablespoon Minced garlic
- 1 ½ teaspoon Salt
- ¾ teaspoon Ground black pepper
- 2 teaspoons Dried rosemary
- 2 teaspoons Dried thyme
- 2 teaspoons Dried oregano
- 2 tablespoons Apple cider vinegar
- 2 tablespoons Avocado oil
- 1 1/2 cups Beef broth, grass-fed

DIRECTIONS

1. Take a frying pan, place it over medium heat, add oil and when hot, add beef and cook for 3 to 5 minutes or until light brown.
2. Transfer beef into a slow cooker, add remaining ingredients, except for spinach and stir until mixed.
3. Switch on the slow cooker, shut it with lid and cook for 5 to 8 hours at low heat setting until thoroughly cooked.
4. When beef cooking is about to finish, place spinach in a heatproof bowl, cover with plastic wrap and microwave for 2 minutes until steamed.
5. When beef is cooked, taste to adjust seasoning, add spinach, and stir until just mixed and let cool.
6. Divide beef evenly between four glass containers, then cover with lid and store in the refrigerator for up to 5 days or freeze for up to 2 months.
7. When ready to serve, thaw the stew at room temperature and then reheat the beef stew in its glass container in the microwave for 2 to 3 minutes or until hot.
8. Serve the stew with cauliflower rice.

NUTRITION

- Calories: 553
- Fat: 36.9g
- Protein: 175g

- Net Carbs: 4.8g
- Fiber: 1.6g

PREPARATION: 10 MIN

COOKING: 12 MIN

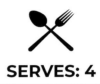
SERVES: 4

COCONUT SHRIMP

INGREDIENTS

- 1 pound Medium-sized shrimp, wild-caught, peeled, deveined
- 3 tablespoons Coconut flour
- 1/4 teaspoon Garlic powder
- 3 Eggs, Pastured, beaten
- 1 3/4 cup Coconut flakes, unsweetened
- 1/8 teaspoon Ground black pepper
- 1/4 teaspoon Smoked paprika
- 1/4 teaspoon Sea salt

DIRECTIONS

1. Set the oven to 400 degrees F and let preheat.
2. Meanwhile, crack eggs in a bowl and whisk until beaten, place coconut flakes in another dish, then place coconut flour in another dish, add salt, black pepper, garlic powder, and paprika and stir until mixed.
3. Working on one piece at a time, dredge a shrimp into the coconut flour mix, then dip into egg, and dredge with coconut flake until evenly coated.
4. Take a non-stick wire rack, line it with a baking sheet, then spray with oil and place coated shrimps on it in a single layer.
5. Place the wire rack containing shrimps into the oven, bake for 4 minutes, then flip the shrimps and continue baking for 5 to 6 minutes or until thoroughly cooked and firm.
6. Then switch on the broiler and bake the shrimps for 2 minutes or until lightly golden.
7. When done, let shrimps cooled, place them on a baking sheet in a single layer, then cover the shrimps with parchment sheet, layer with remaining shrimps and freeze until hard.
8. Then transfer shrimps into a freezer bag and store in the freezer for up to 3 months.
9. When ready to serve, reheat the shrimps at 350 degrees F for 2 to 3 minutes until hot.

NUTRITION

- Calories: 443
- Fat: 30g
- Protein: 31g
- Net Carbs: 5g
- Fiber: 7g

PREPARATION: 10 MIN

COOKING: 1 HOUR

SERVES: 5

CAULIFLOWER RICE SOUP WITH CHICKEN

INGREDIENTS

- 2½ pounds chicken breasts, boneless and skinless
- 8 Tbsp. butter
- ¼ cup celery, chopped
- ½ cup onion, chopped
- 4 cloves garlic, minced
- 2 12-ounce packages steamed cauliflower rice
- 1 Tbsp. parsley, chopped
- 2 tsp. poultry seasoning
- ½ cup carrot, grated
- ¾ tsp. rosemary
- 1 tsp. salt
- ¾ tsp. pepper
- 4 ounces cream cheese
- 4¾ cup chicken broth

DIRECTIONS

1. Put shredded chicken breasts into a saucepan and pour in the chicken broth. Add salt and pepper. Cook for 1 hour.
2. In another pot, melt the butter. Add the onion, garlic, and celery. Sauté until the mix is translucent. Add the rice cauliflower, rosemary, and carrot. Mix and cook for 7 minutes.
3. And then, add the chicken breasts and broth to the cauliflower mix. Put the lid on and simmer for 15 minutes.

NUTRITION

- Carbohydrates: 6g
- Fat: 30g
- Protein: 27g

- Calories: 415

PREPARATION: 10 MIN

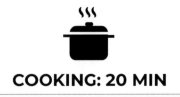

COOKING: 20 MIN

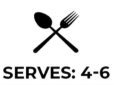

SERVES: 4-6

QUICK PUMPKIN SOUP

INGREDIENTS

- 1 cup of coconut milk
- 2 cups chicken broth
- 6 cups baked pumpkin
- 1 tsp. garlic powder
- 1 tsp. ground cinnamon
- 1 tsp. dried ginger
- 1 tsp. nutmeg
- 1 tsp. paprika Salt and pepper, to taste
- Sour cream or coconut yogurt, for topping
- Pumpkin seeds, toasted, for topping

DIRECTIONS

1. Combine the coconut milk, broth, baked pumpkin, and spices in a soup pan (use medium heat). Stir occasionally and simmer for 15 minutes.
2. With an immersion blender, blend the soup mix for 1 minute.
3. Top with sour cream or coconut yogurt and pumpkin seeds.

NUTRITION

- Carbohydrates: 8.1g
- Fat: 9.8g
- Protein: 3.1g

- Calories: 123

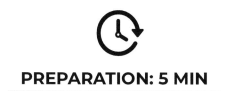

PREPARATION: 5 MIN

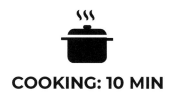

COOKING: 10 MIN

SERVES: 2

FRESH AVOCADO SOUP

INGREDIENTS

- 1 ripe avocado
- 2 romaine lettuce leaves, washed and chopped
- 1 cup coconut milk, chilled
- 1 Tbsp. lime juice
- 20 fresh mint leaves
- Salt, to taste

DIRECTIONS

1. Mix all your ingredients thoroughly in a blender.
2. Chill in the fridge for 5-10 minutes.

NUTRITION

- Carbohydrates: 12g
- Fat: 26g
- Protein: 4g
- Calories: 280

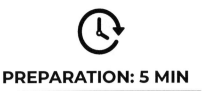

PREPARATION: 5 MIN

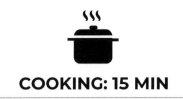

COOKING: 15 MIN

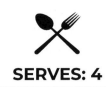

SERVES: 4

CREAMY GARLIC CHICKEN

INGREDIENTS

- 4 chicken breasts, finely sliced
- 1 tsp. garlic powder
- 1 tsp. paprika
- 2 Tbsp. butter
- 1 tsp. salt
- 1 cup heavy cream
- ½ cup sun-dried tomatoes
- 2 cloves garlic, minced
- 1 cup spinach, chopped

DIRECTIONS

1. Blend the paprika, garlic powder, and salt and sprinkle over both sides of the chicken.
2. Melt the butter in a frying pan (choose medium heat). Add the chicken breast and fry for 5 minutes each side. Set aside.
3. Add the heavy cream, sun-dried tomatoes, and garlic to the pan and whisk well to combine. Cook for 2 minutes. Add spinach and sauté for an additional 3 minutes. Return the chicken to the pan and cover with the sauce.

NUTRITION

- Carbohydrates: 12g
- Fat: 26g
- Protein: 4g

- Calories: 280

PREPARATION: 20 MIN

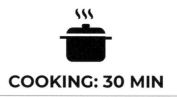

COOKING: 30 MIN

SERVES: 6

CAULIFLOWER CHEESECAKE

INGREDIENTS

- 1 head cauliflower, cut into florets
- 2/3 cup sour cream
- 4 oz. cream cheese softened
- 1½ cup cheddar cheese shredded
- 6 pieces bacon, cooked and chopped
- 1 tsp. salt
- ½ tsp. black pepper
- ¼ cup green onion, chopped
- ¼ tsp. garlic powder

DIRECTIONS

1. Preheat the oven to 350 degrees F.
2. Boil the cauliflower florets for 5 minutes.
3. Then, combine the cream cheese & sour cream in a separate bowl. Mix well and add the cheddar cheese, bacon pieces, green onion, salt, pepper, and garlic powder. Put the cauliflower florets into the bowl and combine with the sauce.
4. Put the cauliflower mix on the baking tray and bake for 15-20 minutes.

NUTRITION

- Carbohydrates: 8g
- Fat: 26g
- Protein: 15g
- Calories: 320

PREPARATION: 5 MIN

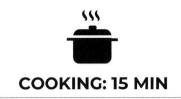

COOKING: 15 MIN

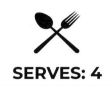

SERVES: 4

CHINESE PORK BOWL

INGREDIENTS

- Salt and ground black pepper, to taste
- 1¼ pounds pork belly, cut into bite-size pieces
- 2 Tbsp. tamari soy sauce
- 1 Tbsp. Rice vinegar
- 2 cloves garlic, smashed
- 3 oz. butter
- 1 pound Brussels sprouts, rinsed, trimmed, halved or quartered
- ½ leek, chopped

DIRECTIONS

1. Fry the pork over medium-high heat until it is starting to turn golden brown.
2. Combine the garlic cloves, butter, and Brussels sprouts. Add to the pan, whisk well and cook until the sprouts turn golden brown.
3. Stir the soy sauce & rice vinegar together and pour the sauce into the pan.
4. Sprinkle with salt and pepper.
5. Top with chopped leek.

NUTRITION

- Carbohydrates: 7g
- Fat: 97g
- Protein: 19g

- Calories: 993

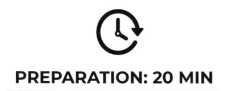

PREPARATION: 20 MIN

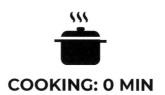

COOKING: 0 MIN

SERVES: 1

TURKEY-PEPPER MIX

INGREDIENTS

- 1 pound turkey tenderloin, cut into thin steaks
- 1 tsp. salt, divided
- 2 Tbsp. extra-virgin olive oil, divided
- ½ sweet onion, sliced
- 1 red bell pepper, cut into strips
- 1 yellow bell pepper, cut into strips
- ½ tsp. Italian seasoning
- ¼ tsp. ground black pepper
- 2 tsp. red wine vinegar
- 1 14-ounces crushed tomatoes, roasted Fresh parsley Basil

DIRECTIONS

1. Sprinkle ½ tsp. salt on your turkey. Pour 1 Tbsp. Oil into the pan and heat it. Add the turkey steaks and cook for 1-3 minutes per side. Set aside.
2. Put the onion, bell peppers, and the remaining salt to the pan and cook for 7 minutes, stirring all the time. Sprinkle with Italian seasoning and add black pepper. Cook for 30 seconds. Add the tomatoes and vinegar and fry the mix for about 20 seconds.
3. Now, return the turkey to the pan & pour the sauce over it. Simmer for 2-3 minutes.
4. Top with chopped parsley and basil.

NUTRITION

- Carbohydrates: 11g
- Fat: 8g
- Protein: 30g

- Calories: 230

12. DRINKS

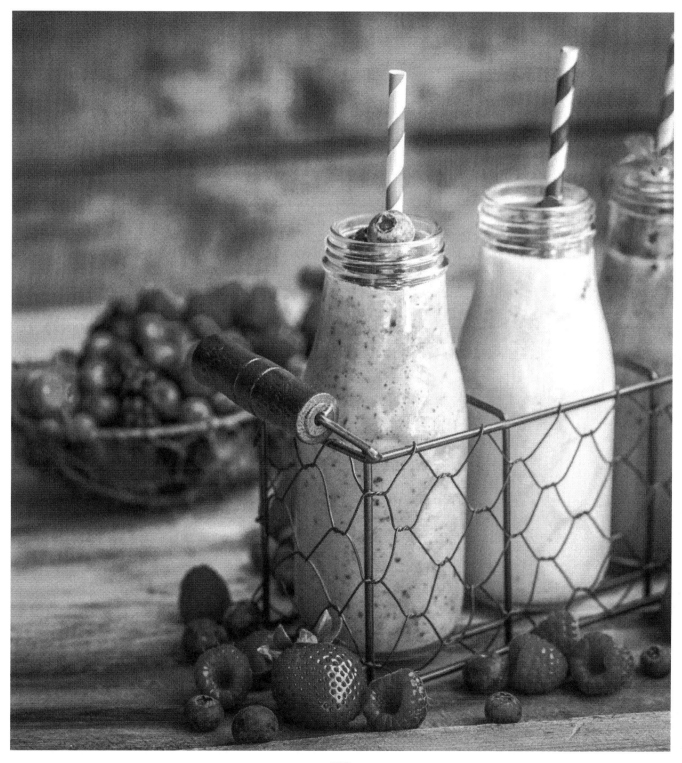

PREPARATION: 10 MIN

COOKING: 10 MIN

SERVES: 2

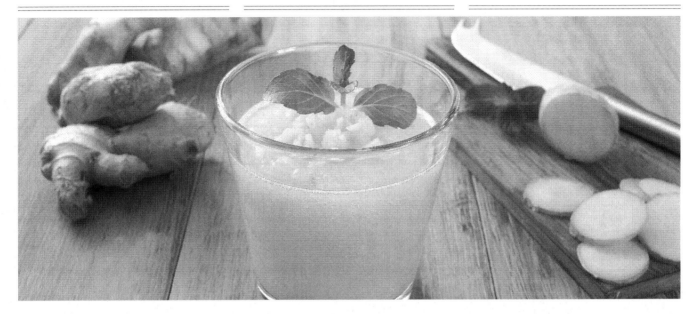

BRACING GINGER SMOOTHIE

INGREDIENTS

- ⅓ Cup coconut cream
- ⅔ Cup water
- 2 tablespoons lime juice
- 1 oz. spinach, frozen
- 2 tablespoons ginger, grated

DIRECTIONS

1. Blend all the ingredients. Add 1 tablespoon lime at first and increase the amount if necessary.
2. Top with grated ginger and enjoy your smoothie!

NUTRITION

- Calories: 82
- Fat: 8grams
- Net Carbs: 3grams

- Protein: 1gram

PREPARATION: 5 MIN

COOKING: 10 MIN

SERVES: 1

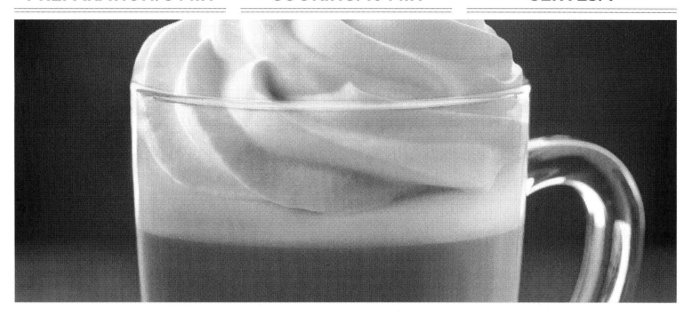

MORNING COFFEE WITH CREAM

INGREDIENTS

- ¾ cup coffee
- ¼ cup whipping cream

DIRECTIONS

1. Make your favorite coffee.
2. Pour the heavy cream in a small saucepan and heat slowly until you get a frothy texture.
3. Pour the hot cream in a big cup, add coffee and enjoy your morning drink.

NUTRITION

- Calories: 202
- Fat: 21grams
- Net Carbs: 2grams
- Protein: 2grams

PREPARATION: 5 MIN

COOKING: 0 MIN

SERVES: 2

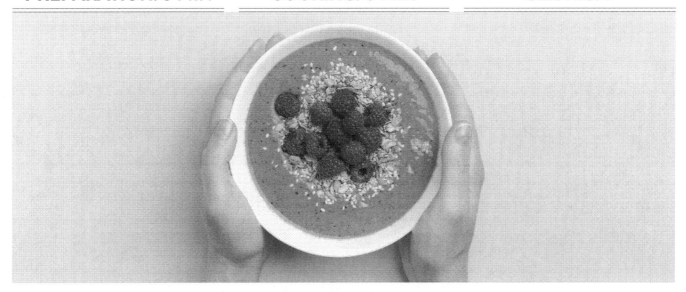

BERRY BLAST SMOOTHIE

INGREDIENTS

- 2 cups fresh spinach
- ½ cup frozen mixed berries (such as blueberries, raspberries, and strawberries)
- 2 tablespoons hemp seeds
- Half of an avocado, ripe
- 1 cup water

DIRECTIONS

1. Add the entire ingredients in a blender and blend on high power until completely smooth and creamy.

NUTRITION

- Calories: 164
- Total Fat: 12g
- Saturated Fat: 1.6g
- Total Carbohydrates: 12g
- Dietary Fiber: 5.4g
- Sugar: 4.3g
- Protein: 5.3g

PREPARATION: 5 MIN

COOKING: 0 MIN

SERVES: 2

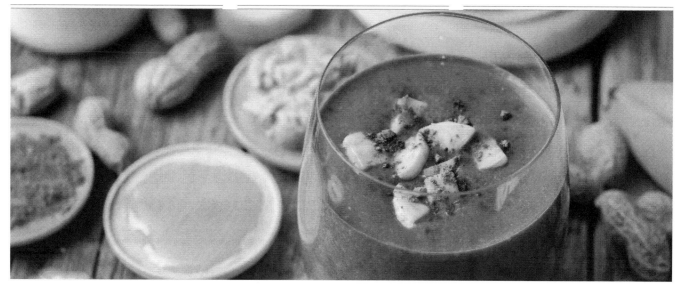

CHOCOLATE PEANUT BUTTER SMOOTHIE

INGREDIENTS

- 1 tablespoon unsweetened cocoa powder
- 2 tablespoons creamy peanut butter
- 1 cup unsweetened almond milk or any plant-based milk, low-carb
- ¼ cup heavy cream
- 1 cup crushed ice

DIRECTIONS

1. Add the entire ingredients in a blender and blend on high power until completely smooth and creamy.

NUTRITION

- Calories: 268
- Total Fat: 21g
- Saturated Fat: 9.8.g
- Total Carbohydrates: 6g

- Dietary Fiber: 1.4g
- Sugars: 1.9g
- Protein: 9.1g

PREPARATION: 5 MIN

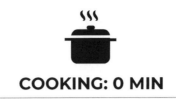

COOKING: 0 MIN

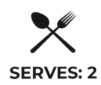

SERVES: 2

LOW-CARB STRAWBERRY SMOOTHIE

INGREDIENTS

- ¾ cup almond milk, unsweetened
- 4 oz. strawberries, frozen
- ¼ cup coconut cream or heavy whipping cream
- 2 teaspoons erythritol blend or granulated stevia
- ½ teaspoon vanilla extract
- ½ cup ice, optional

DIRECTIONS

1. Add the entire ingredients together (with the optional ice) in a blender and blend until completely smooth and creamy, on high power.

NUTRITION

- Calories: 168
- Total Fat: 7.1g
- Saturated Fat: 5.8g
- Total Carbohydrates: 6g

- Dietary Fiber: 3.5g
- Sugars: 3.5g
- Protein: 1.1g

PREPARATION: 5 MIN

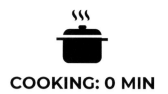

COOKING: 0 MIN

SERVES: 2

BLUEBERRY SMOOTHIE

INGREDIENTS

- 1 cup coconut milk
- 1 teaspoon vanilla extract
- ¼ cup fresh blueberries
- 1 teaspoon coconut oil or MCT oil
- 1 scoop protein powder, optional

DIRECTIONS

1. Add all of the ingredients together in a blender and blend on high power until completely smooth and creamy.

NUTRITION

- Calories: 260
- Total Fat: 26g
- Saturated Fat: 23g
- Total Carbohydrates: 6.1g
- Dietary Fiber: 0.4g
- Sugars: 2.1g
- Protein: 5.6g

PREPARATION: 5 MIN

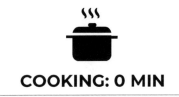

COOKING: 0 MIN

SERVES: 2

CINNAMON RASPBERRY BREAKFAST SMOOTHIE

INGREDIENTS

- ½ cup raspberries, frozen
- 1 cup unsweetened almond milk
- 2 tablespoons almond butter
- 1 cup spinach or kale
- 1/8 teaspoon cinnamon, to taste

DIRECTIONS

1. Add the entire ingredients together in a blender and blend until completely smooth and creamy, on high power.

NUTRITION

- Calories: 136
- Total Fat: 10.3g
- Saturated Fat: 0.9g
- Total Carbohydrates: 8.3g

- Dietary Fiber: 4.1g
- Sugars: 3.2g
- Protein: 4.7g

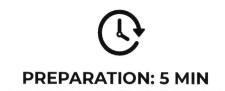
PREPARATION: 5 MIN

COOKING: 5 MIN

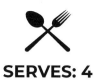
SERVES: 4

CREAMY HOT CHOCOLATE

INGREDIENTS

- 6 oz. dark chocolate, chopped
- ½ cup unsweetened almond milk
- ½ cup heavy cream
- 1 Tbsp. erythritol
- ½ tsp. vanilla extract

DIRECTIONS

1. Combine the almond milk, erythritol, and cream in a small saucepan. Heat it (choose medium heat and cook for 1-2 minutes).
2. Add vanilla extract and chocolate. Stir continuously until the chocolate melts.
3. Pour into cups and serve.

NUTRITION

- Carbohydrates: 4g
- Fat: 18g
- Protein: 2g
- Calories: 193

13. SIDES

PREPARATION: 15 MIN

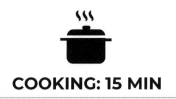

COOKING: 15 MIN

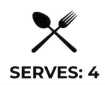

SERVES: 4

ALMOND FLOUR CRACKERS

INGREDIENTS

- 1 tablespoon flax meal or whole Psyllium husks
- 2 tablespoons sunflower seeds
- 1 cup almond flour
- 2 tablespoons water
- 1 tablespoon coconut oil
- ¾ teaspoon sea salt or to taste

DIRECTIONS

1. Preheat your oven to 350°F.
2. Blend the almond flour with Psyllium, sunflower seeds and sea salt in a food processor or large bowl.
3. If you are blending the ingredients by hand then stir the liquid ingredients into dry ingredients to form a dough ball or if you are using a food processor then pulse in coconut oil and water until dough forms.
4. Place the formed ball of dough on a parchment paper; pressing it flat. Cover with one more parchment paper; rolling the dough out to approximately 1/8 to 1/16" thickness.
5. Put it on a large cutting board; remove the parchment paper on top and cut into 1" squares using a pizza cutter or sharp knife. Sprinkle with the sea salt.
6. Place the cut dough on a large-sized baking sheet; bake in a 350°F oven for 10 to 15 minutes, until edges are crisp and brown. Let cool on a rack and then separate into desired squares.

NUTRITION

- Calories: 149
- Total Fat: 13g
- Saturated Fat: 2.8g
- Total Carbohydrates: 4.7g
- Dietary Fiber: 2.9g
- Sugars: 0.9g
- Protein: 4.7g

PREPARATION: 10 MIN

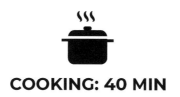
COOKING: 40 MIN

SERVES: 6

GLUTEN-FREE BAGELS

INGREDIENTS

- 1 teaspoon baking powder
- ¼ cup Psyllium husks
- ½ cup tahini
- 1 cup water
- ½ cup ground flaxseed
- Sesame seeds for garnish, optional

DIRECTIONS

1. Preheat your oven to 375°F in advance.
2. Add the Psyllium husk together with baking powder and ground flaxseeds to a large-sized mixing bowl; whisk until combined well.
3. Add water to the tahini; continue to whisk until combined well.
4. Stir the dry ingredients into the wet; knead until dough ball forms.
5. Form approximately 4" diameter and ¼" thick patties from the prepared batter using your hands. Arrange them on the prepared baking tray and cut a small circle from the center of each round.
6. Sprinkle sesame seeds on the patties.
7. Bake in the preheated oven until turn golden brown, for 35 to 40 minutes.
8. Cut in half and toast just like you do for a normal bagel and then top with your favorite toppings.

NUTRITION

- Calories: 215
- Total Fat: 16g
- Saturated Fat: 2.2g
- Total Carbohydrates: 14g
- Dietary Fiber: 12.1g
- Sugars: 0.2g
- Protein: 6g

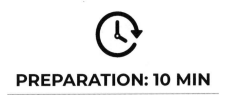

PREPARATION: 10 MIN

COOKING: 30 MIN

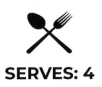

SERVES: 4

ROASTED CABBAGE WITH LEMON

INGREDIENTS

- 2-3 tablespoons lemon juice, freshly squeezed
- 1/2 head of green cabbage, cut into 8 evenly size wedges, cutting it through the core and stem end
- Fresh ground black pepper and sea salt to taste
- 2 tablespoons olive oil
- Lemon slices, for serving

DIRECTIONS

1. Lightly coat a roasting pan with the olive oil or non-stick spray and then preheat your oven to 450°F.
2. Arrange the cabbage wedges on the prepared roasting pan, preferably in a single layer.
3. Whisk the olive oil with lemon juice then brush the top sides of each wedge with the prepared mixture using a pastry brush and generously season with fresh ground black pepper and salt.
4. Carefully turn the cabbage wedges and brush the other side with the lemon juice-olive oil mixture as well then season with pepper and salt.
5. Roast the cabbage until the sides of your wedges is nicely browned, for 12 to 15 minutes.
6. Remove the pan from oven; carefully turning the wedges. Put in the oven again and roast until the cabbage is cooked through and nicely browned, for 10 to 15 more minutes.
7. Serve hot with more of lemon slices, if desired.

NUTRITION

- Calories: 129
- Total Fat: 7.6g
- Saturated Fat: 1.1g
- Total Carbohydrates: 8.5g
- Dietary Fiber: 3g
- Sugars: 4.5g
- Protein: 2g

PREPARATION: 5 MIN   **COOKING: 0 + 30 MIN REFRIGERATED**   **SERVES: 6**

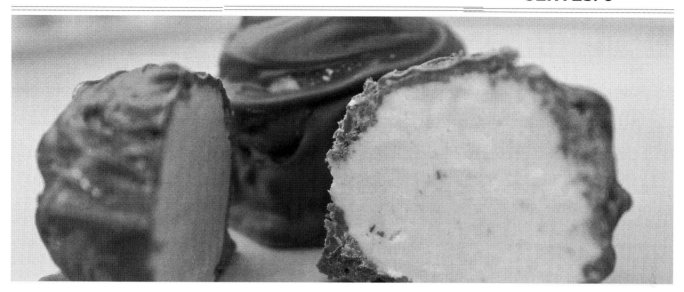

KETO PEANUT BUTTER BALLS

INGREDIENTS

- 1/3 cup coconut flour
- ¼ cup smooth peanut butter
- ¼ cup monk fruit sweetened maple syrup

DIRECTIONS

1. Line a large-sized plate or tray with parchment paper in advance; set aside until ready to use.
2. Now, combine the entire ingredients together in a large-sized mixing bowl; mix well. If the batter appears to be too thick, immediately add a small amount of water (but ensure that the batter still remains thick).
3. Form the dough into small balls using your hands; placing each ball on the lined tray or plate. Refrigerate until firm, for 30 minutes.

NUTRITION

- Calories: 132
- Total Fat: 6.6g
- Saturated Fat: 1.8g
- Total Carbohydrates: 6.4g

- Dietary Fiber: 5.5g
- Sugars: 1.2g
- Protein: 3.5g

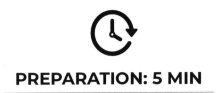
PREPARATION: 5 MIN

COOKING: 15 MIN

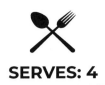
SERVES: 4

SPINACH-MOZZARELLA STUFFED BURGERS

INGREDIENTS

- 1 pounds ground chuck
- 2 tablespoons Parmesan cheese, grated
- ½ cup mozzarella cheese, shredded (approximately 4 oz.)
- 2 cups firmly packed spinach, fresh
- ¾ teaspoon ground black pepper
- 1 teaspoon salt

DIRECTIONS

1. Combine the ground beef together with pepper and salt in a medium-sized bowl.
2. Scoop approximately ⅓ cup of the prepared mixture and shape into 8 approximately ½" thick patties using dampened hands. Place in a refrigerator until ready to use.
3. Now, over medium-high heat in a large saucepan; add the spinach. Cover and cook until wilted, for 2 minutes.
4. Drain and let cool. Squeeze the spinach and extract the liquid as much as possible using your hands.
5. Transfer to a clean, large cutting board; chop the spinach and place in a large-sized bowl.
6. Stir in Parmesan and mozzarella cheese. Scoop approximately ¼ cup of the stuffing and mound in middle of 4 patties.
7. Cover with the leftover patties; press firmly and seal the edges. Using your hands; cup each patty to round out the edges; pressing on the top to slightly flattens into a thick patty.
8. Heat a grill pan or grill over medium-high heat. Grill the burgers for 3 to 5 minutes per side. Serve immediately and enjoy.

NUTRITION

- Calories: 323
- Total Fat: 15.8g
- Saturated Fat: 8.1g
- Total Carbohydrates: 1.6g

- Dietary Fiber: 0.3g
- Sugars: 0.4g
- Protein: 41.7g

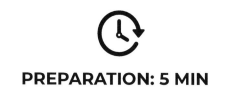

PREPARATION: 5 MIN

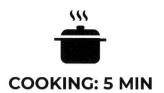

COOKING: 5 MIN

SERVES: 12

AVOCADO TUNA MELT BITES

INGREDIENTS

- .25 cup Mayo
- .25 cup Parmesan cheese
- 10 oz. can Drained tuna
- .33 cup Almond flour
- .25 tsp. Onion powder
- Pepper and salt (to your liking)
- .5 tsp. Garlic powder
- 1 medium Cubed avocado
- 2 tbsp. To Fry: Coconut oil

DIRECTIONS

1. Combine all of the fixings in a bowl—omitting the oil and avocado for now.
2. Fold in the tuna with the cubed avocado. Shape into balls and coat with the flour.
3. Heat the oil using the medium-temperature setting and fry until golden brown to serve.

NUTRITION

- Calories: 185
- Net Carbohydrates: 1g
- Protein: 5g
- Fat Content: 17.8g

PREPARATION: 5 MIN

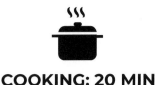
COOKING: 20 MIN

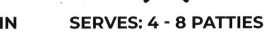
SERVES: 4 - 8 PATTIES

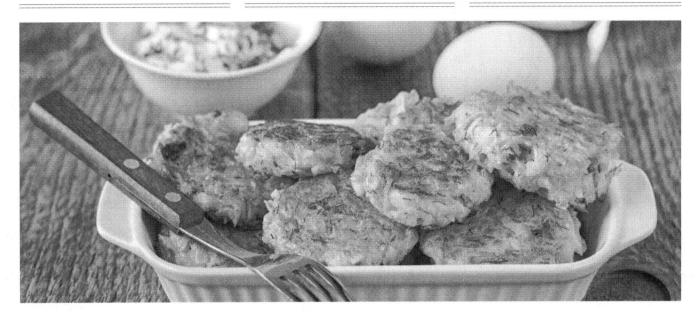

CABBAGE PATTIES

INGREDIENTS

- 3 cups Cabbage, or 1 large Egg
- .75 tbsp Coconut flour
- 2 tbsp Coconut oil, melted
- Optional: Garlic powder & salt

DIRECTIONS

1. Cook and finely chop the cabbage. Toss it with the seasonings and flour into a food processor. Pulse three to four times or until the coconut flour is evenly dispersed.
2. Crack the egg into the mixture and add the oil. Pulse it for another three to four pulses to combine thoroughly. Don't the cabbage too fine.
3. Roll the mixture into eight balls and flatten.
4. Lightly spray a skillet with a cooking oil spray or add additional fat. Add the patties and cook until done.
5. Serve the patties plain or top it off as desired—but count the carbs.

NUTRITION

- Net Carbohydrates: 1g
- Fat Content: 4g
- Protein: 1g

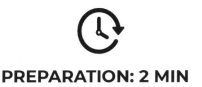
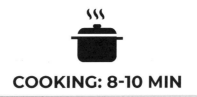

COOL & SPICY JICAMA SLAW

INGREDIENTS

- 200g/4 cups Julienned jicama
- 200g/1 large Avocado
- 200g/4 cups Julienned cucumber
- 50g/2 large Radish, sliced thinly
- 25g/2 tbsp. Grape seed oil
- 25g/2 tbsp. Lime juice
- Optional: Red chili pepper flakes (as desired)

DIRECTIONS

1. Use the widest julienne setting to prepare the jicama and cucumber. Weigh or measure, and combine them in a large mixing container.
2. Use the thinnest setting to slice the radish and toss them with the cucs.
3. Prepare the juice by squeezing the lime and straining any seeds from the juice. Dice the avocado and toss in the juice until coated to help prevent the avocado from premature browning.
4. Toss the avocado with the veggies.
5. If you prefer a creamier slaw, mash the avocado with the juice until smooth, and add the avocado mixture to the jicama. Pour the oil over the mixture, tossing to combine.
6. If using, mix in the chili flakes and wait about ½ hour before serving.

NUTRITION

- Net Carbohydrates: 3g
- Fat Content: 7g
- Protein: 1g

PREPARATION: 10 MIN

COOKING: 20-25 MIN

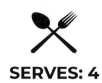

SERVES: 4

CREAMY GREEN CABBAGE

INGREDIENTS

- 2 oz. Butter
- 1.5 lb. Shredded green cabbage
- 1.25 cups Coconut cream
- 8 tbsp. Finely chopped fresh parsley
- Pepper and salt (as desired)

DIRECTIONS

1. Shred the cabbage and add to a skillet with the butter. Sauté until its golden brown.
2. Stir in the cream with a sprinkle of salt and pepper. Simmer.
3. Garnish with the parsley and serve while warm.

PREPARATION: 10 MIN

COOKING: 35-40 MIN

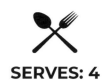

SERVES: 4

CREAMY SPINACH-RICH BALLET

INGREDIENTS

- 1.5 lb. Fresh baby spinach
- 8 tsp. Coconut cream
- 14 oz. Sliced cauliflower
- 2 tbsp. Melted-unsalted butter
- Black pepper and salt (to your liking)
- Also Needed: 4 ramekins

DIRECTIONS

1. Set the oven temperature at 360° Fahrenheit.
2. Prepare a skillet with the butter. Toss in the spinach to sauté for three minutes.
3. Drain the juices from the spinach and add to the ramekins.
4. Slice the cauliflower and add to the containers with the cream, salt, and pepper.
5. Bake for 25 minutes. Enjoy it warm.

NUTRITION

- Calories: 188
- Net Carbohydrates: 2.9g
- Protein: 14.6g
- Fat Content: 12.5g

PREPARATION: 20 MIN

COOKING: 2 HOURS

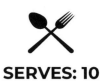
SERVES: 10

DRIED BEEF & CREAM CHEESE BALL

INGREDIENTS

- 8 oz. Shredded cheddar cheese
- 3 oz. Cream cheese
- .5 tsp. Worcestershire sauce
- .25 cup Black olives
- Salt: Celery, Garlic & Onion salt (1 pinch each)
- 4 oz. jar Dried beef

DIRECTIONS

1. Chop the dried beef and set aside.
2. Combine the rest of the fixings. Mix until smooth.
3. Shape into a ball and roll through the beef.
4. Arrange them on a piece of aluminum foil.
5. Refrigerate until ready to serve. Chill overnight or for several hours.

NUTRITION

- Calories: 143
- Net Carbohydrates: 1.1g
- Protein: 10g

- Fat Content: 11g

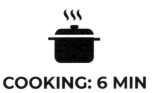
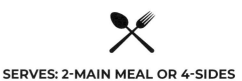
GARLIC & OLIVE OIL SPAGHETTI SQUASH

INGREDIENTS

- 1 Spaghetti squash
- 3-4 Garlic cloves
- 2 tbsp Olive oil
- .25 cup Water
- Salt and pepper (to your liking)

DIRECTIONS

1. Warm the oven to reach 375° Fahrenheit.
2. Slice the squash in half—lengthwise. Scoop out seeds, saving as much of the inside as possible.
3. Prepare a casserole with a bit of cooking oil spray. Place the squash face-down, and add the water.
4. Bake for ½ hour. Flip the squash and continue cooking for an additional ½ hour—until softened.
5. Mince and sauté the garlic and add the oil in a pan.
6. Grab a serving fork to scrape the squash into the pan. Add the garlic and olive oil.
7. Cook for another three to five minutes with a shake of pepper and salt.

NUTRITION

- Calories: 181.4
- Net Carbohydrates: 11.6g
- Protein: 1.7g

- Fat Content: 14.5g

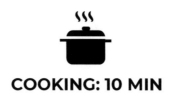

MARINARA ZOODLES

INGREDIENTS

- 2 tbsp E-V olive oil
- 6 Garlic cloves
- .5 cup White onions
- 14 oz. diced Tomatoes
- 2 tbsp. Tomato paste
- .5 cup Basil leaves, roughly-chopped, loosely packed)
- 1.5 tsp. Coarse salt
- .25 tsp Freshly cracked black pepper
- 1 pinch Cayenne
- 2 Large zucchini, spiralizer

DIRECTIONS

1. Add the oil to the skillet before placing it on the stovetop (medium-temperature setting).
2. Mince the onion and garlic. Toss them in and sauté the onion for about five minutes before adding in the garlic. Cook for approximately one minute.
3. Mix in the salt, crushed red pepper flakes, pepper, salt, basil, tomato paste, and tomatoes. Combine thoroughly.
4. Simmer the sauce and lower the temperature setting to medium-low. Simmer an additional 15 minutes or until the oil takes on a deep orange color which indicates the sauce is thickened and reduced. Season as desired.
5. Add in the Zoodles and let them soften approximately two minutes before serving.

NUTRITION

- Calories: 179
- Net Carbohydrates: 5.1g
- Protein: 7g
- Fat Content: 19g

PREPARATION: 10 MIN

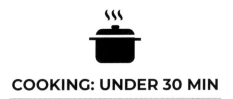

COOKING: UNDER 30 MIN

SERVES: 4

MUSHROOM & CAULIFLOWER RISOTTO

INGREDIENTS

- 1 Grated head of cauliflower
- 1 cup Vegetable stock
- 9 oz Chopped mushrooms
- 2 tbsp Butter
- 1 cup Coconut cream
- Pepper and Salt (to taste)

DIRECTIONS

1. Pour the stock in a saucepan. Boil and set aside.
2. Prepare a skillet with butter and sauté the mushrooms until golden.
3. Grate and stir in the cauliflower and stock.
4. Simmer and add the cream, cooking until the cauliflower is al dente to serve.

NUTRITION

- Calories: 186
- Net Carbohydrates: 4.3g
- Fat Content: 17.1g

PREPARATION: 10 MIN

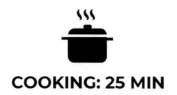

COOKING: 25 MIN

SERVES: 4

RED PEPPER ZOODLES

INGREDIENTS

- 1 Garlic clove
- 1 Red bell peppers
- 1 cup Almond milk
- 1 tbsp. Olive oil
- 1 tsp. Salt
- .25 cup Almond butter

DIRECTIONS

1. Prepare a baking sheet by lining it with foil.
2. Add the bell peppers to the baking sheet before placing them on the top level of your broiler and letting them cook until blackened. Remove and cool.
3. Once they have cooled you can remove the skins, stems, seeds, and ribs.
4. Add the prepared mixture, along with the remaining sauce ingredients, and blend thoroughly. Season as desired.
5. Serve with Zoodles as well as a variety of potential toppings including things like truffle oil, goat cheese, or parsley.

NUTRITION

- Calories: 198
- Net Carbohydrates: 4.1g
- Protein: 5g

- Fat Content: 16.7g

PREPARATION: 10 MIN

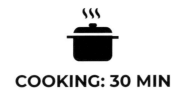

COOKING: 30 MIN

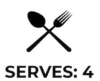

SERVES: 4

STUFFED MUSHROOMS

INGREDIENTS

- 4 Portobello mushrooms
- 1 cup Blue cheese
- 2 tbsp Olive oil
- 1 pinch Fresh thyme
- Salt (as desired)

DIRECTIONS

1. Set the oven temperature at 350° Fahrenheit.
2. Cut the stems from the mushrooms and chop them to bits.
3. Mix with the thyme, salt, and crumbled blue cheese and stuff the mushrooms.
4. Spritz with some of the oil.
5. Bake for 15-20 minutes.
6. Serve it piping hot.

NUTRITION

- Calories: 124
- Net Carbohydrates: 2.6g
- Protein: 5g
- Fat Content: 22.4g

PREPARATION: 45 MIN

COOKING: 1 3/4 HOUR

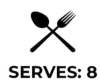

SERVES: 8

ZUCCHINI NOODLE GRATIN

INGREDIENTS

- 8 cups/800g Loosely packed zucchini noodles
- 1 cup/238g Heavy cream
- 4 oz./113g Shredded Gruyere cheese
- 3 tbsp./42g Butter
- Optional Seasonings:
- Black pepper
- Salt
- Garlic powder
- Fresh herbs
- Also Needed: 9-inch baking dish

DIRECTIONS

1. Make the zucchini noodles and place them in a mesh colander. Grab and garnish using the salt and toss to coat evenly. Leave them in the sink for about two hours to release moisture. Gently dry and squeeze the excess moisture from the noodles with a paper towel.
2. Warm the oven to reach 350° Fahrenheit. Lightly grease the baking dish with butter and add the noodles in an even layer.
3. Use a saucepan to combine the butter, heavy cream, and cheese. Warm the mixture using the medium-temperature setting until melted and the sauce is smooth. Transfer the pan to a cool burner and add optional seasonings.
4. Pour the cream mixture over the noodles and bake for about one hour or until nicely browned.
5. Cool the gratin for about 15 minutes and slice into eight portions to serve.

NUTRITION

- Calories: 200
- Net Carbohydrates: 3g
- Protein: 6g

- Fat Content: 18g

14. MEAT

PREPARATION: 5 MIN

COOKING: 20 MIN

SERVES: 2

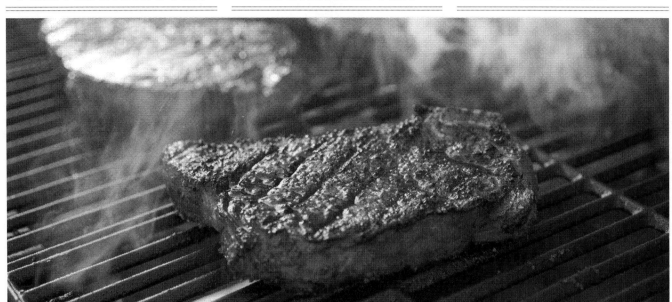

KETO RIB EYE STEAK

INGREDIENTS

- ½ pound grass-fed rib-eye steak, preferably 1" thick
- 1 teaspoon Adobo Seasoning
- 1 tablespoon extra-virgin olive oil
- Pepper and sea salt to taste

DIRECTIONS

1. Add steak in a large-sized mixing bowl and drizzle both sides with a small amount of olive oil. Dust the seasonings on both sides; rubbing the seasonings into the meat.
2. Let sit for a couple of minutes and heat up your grill in advance. Once hot; place the steaks over the grill, and cook until both sides are cooked through, for 15 to 20 minutes, flipping occasionally.

NUTRITION

- Calories: 258 Cal
- Fat: 19g
- Carbs: 5g

- Protein: 8g
- Fiber: 8g

PREPARATION: 5 MIN

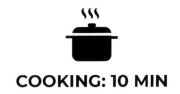

COOKING: 10 MIN

SERVES: 2

KETO GROUND BEEF AND GREEN BEANS

INGREDIENTS

- 1 ½ oz. butter
- 8 ozs. green beans, fresh, rinsed, and trimmed
- 10 ozs. ground beef
- 1/4 cup Crème Fraiche or home-made mayonnaise, optional
- Pepper and salt to taste

DIRECTIONS

1. Over moderate heat in a large, frying pan; heat a generous dollop of butter until completely melted.
2. Increase the heat to high and immediately brown the ground beef until almost done, for 5 minutes. Sprinkle with pepper and salt to taste.
3. Decrease the heat to medium; add more of butter and continue to fry the beans in the same pan with the meat for 5 more minutes, stirring frequently.
4. Season the beans with pepper and salt as well. Serve with the leftover butter and add in the optional Crème Fraiche or mayonnaise, if desired.

NUTRITION

- Calories: 238 Cal
- Fat: 15g
- Carbs: 8g
- Protein: 10g
- Fiber: 4g

PREPARATION: 10 MIN

COOKING: 10 MIN

SERVES: 3

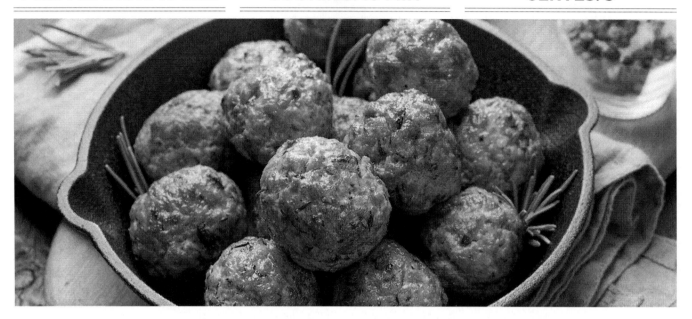

SPICY BEEF MEATBALLS

INGREDIENTS

- 1 cup mozzarella or cheddar cheese; cut into 1x1 cm cubes
- 1 pound minced ground beef
- 1 teaspoon olive oil
- 3 tablespoons parmesan cheese
- 1 teaspoon garlic powder
- ½ teaspoon each of pepper, and salt

DIRECTIONS

1. Thoroughly combine the ground beef with the entire dry ingredients; mix well.
2. Wrap the cheese cubes into the mince; forming 9 meatballs from the prepared mixture.
3. Pan-fry the formed meatballs until cooked through, covered (uncover and stirring frequently).

NUTRITION

- Calories: 358 Cal
- Fat: 19g
- Carbs: 4g

- Protein: 18g
- Fiber: 5g

PREPARATION: 15 MIN

COOKING: 10 MIN

SERVES: 6

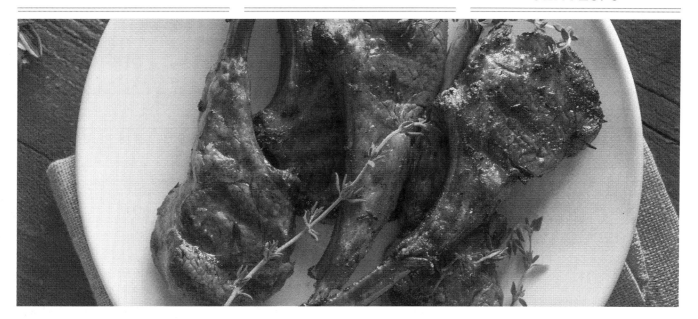

GARLIC & THYME LAMB CHOPS

INGREDIENTS

- 6-4 oz. Lamb chops
- 4 whole garlic cloves
- 2 thyme sprigs
- 1 tsp. Ground thyme
- 3 tbsp. Olive oil

DIRECTIONS

1. Warm-up a skillet. Put the olive oil. Rub the chops with the spices.
2. Put the chops in the skillet with the garlic and sprigs of thyme.
3. Sauté within 3 to 4 minutes and serve.

NUTRITION

- Net Carbohydrates: 1gram
- Protein: 14grams
- Total Fats: 21grams
- Calories: 252

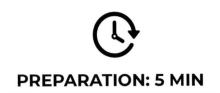
PREPARATION: 5 MIN

COOKING: 4 HOURS

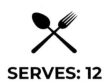
SERVES: 12

JAMAICAN JERK PORK ROAST

INGREDIENTS

- 1 tbsp. Olive oil
- 4 lb. Pork shoulder
- .5 cup Beef Broth
- .25 cup Jamaican Jerk spice blend

DIRECTIONS

1. Rub the roast well the oil and the jerk spice blend. Sear the roast on all sides. Put the beef broth.
2. Simmer within four hours on low. Shred and serve.

NUTRITION

- Net Carbohydrates: 0grams
- Protein: 23grams
- Total Fats: 20grams
- Calories: 282

PREPARATION: 15 MIN

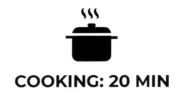

COOKING: 20 MIN

SERVES: 10

KETO MEATBALLS

INGREDIENTS

- 1 egg
- .5 cup Grated parmesan
- .5 cup Shredded mozzarella
- 1 lb. Ground beef
- 1 tbsp. garlic

DIRECTIONS

1. Warm-up the oven to reach 400. Combine all of the fixings.
2. Shape into meatballs. Bake within 18-20 minutes. Cool and serve.

NUTRITION

- Net Carbohydrates: 0.7grams
- Protein: 12.2grams
- Total Fats: 10.9grams
- Calories: 153

PREPARATION: 15 MIN

COOKING: 1H 30 MIN

SERVES: 6

ROASTED LEG OF LAMB

INGREDIENTS

- .5 cup Reduced-sodium beef broth
- 2 lb. lamb leg
- 6garlic cloves
- 1 tbsp. rosemary leaves
- 1 tsp. Black pepper

DIRECTIONS

1. Warm-up oven temperature to 400 Fahrenheit.
2. Put the lamb in the pan and put the broth and seasonings.
3. Roast 30 minutes and lower the heat to 350° Fahrenheit. Cook within one hour.
4. Cool and serve.

NUTRITION

- Net Carbohydrates: 1gram
- Protein: 22grams
- Total Fats: 14grams

- Calories: 223

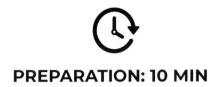
PREPARATION: 10 MIN

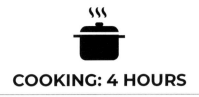
COOKING: 4 HOURS

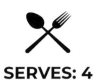
SERVES: 4

FLAVORFUL PULLED PORK

INGREDIENTS

- 2 lbs. pork shoulder
- 1/3 cup chicken broth
- 1 ½ teaspoon cocoa powder
- ½ teaspoon ground fennel seeds
- ½ teaspoon cayenne
- 1 ½ teaspoons paprika
- 2 teaspoons dried rosemary
- 1 teaspoon garlic powder
- 2 teaspoons onion powder
- ¼ teaspoon pepper
- 1 tablespoon of sea salt

DIRECTIONS

1. In a small bowl, mix together cocoa powder and all spices.
2. Rub spice mixture over pork shoulder. Place pork shoulder in the slow cooker.
3. Pour broth over pork shoulder.
4. Cover slow cooker with lid
5. And cook on high for 4 hours.
6. Remove pork from slow cooker and shred using a fork.
7. Serve and enjoy.

NUTRITION

- Calories: 679
- Fat: 49grams
- Net Carbs: 3grams
- Protein: 53.8grams

PREPARATION: 25 MIN

COOKING: 10 MIN

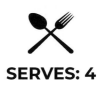
SERVES: 4

ITALIAN LAMB CHOPS

INGREDIENTS

- 8 lamb chops
- 2 tablespoons olive oil
- 2 tablespoons Dijon mustard
- 1 ½ teaspoon Italian seasoning
- 1 teaspoon garlic, minced
- Pepper
- Salt

DIRECTIONS

1. Preheat the oven to 425°F.
2. Season pork chops with pepper and salt and place on a baking tray.
3. In a small bowl, mix together the remaining ingredients and spoon over each pork chops and spread well.
4. Bake for 15 minutes.
5. Serve and enjoy.

NUTRITION

- Calories: 391
- Fat: 21.2grams
- Net Carbs: 1gram

- Protein: 48grams

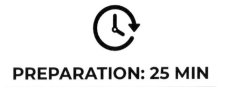

PREPARATION: 25 MIN

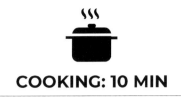

COOKING: 10 MIN

SERVES: 4

QUICK AND EASY MONGOLIAN BEEF

INGREDIENTS

- 1 pound flank steak thinly sliced against the grain
- 2 tablespoons cornstarch
- 2-4 tablespoons canola oil
- 1 yellow onion sliced
- 2 green onions chopped, green and white parts separated
- 4 garlic cloves chopped
- 1/4 c. low sodium soy sauce
- 1/4 c. water
- 1 tablespoon hoisin sauce
- 3 tablespoons brown sugar
- Add salt to taste

DIRECTIONS

1. Cover with cornstarch the flank steak, ensuring that each slice is coated.
2. Heat the canola oil over medium to high heat in a large skillet. When the oil is heated, apply the flank steak in a single layer to the frying pan, making sure that the parts do not touch. Cook until each surface is browned, for 1-2 minutes per surface. Cook until all the flank steak is finished, in batches.
3. Apply the sliced yellow onion, green onion whites, garlic, and ginger to the skillet and fry for around three minutes, until the onions are somewhat softened but still crunchy. Apply soy sauce, water, brown sugar, and hoisin sauce and stir. Along with the green sections of the onions, add the steak back to the plate. Withdraw from the heat and serve.

NUTRITION

- Calories: 303
- Fat: 13g (3g sat)
- Protein: 26g
- Carb: 20g

- Sodium: 670mg
- Sugars: 11g
- Fiber: 1g

PREPARATION: 25 MIN

COOKING: 10 MIN

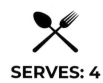

SERVES: 4

BEEF NOODLE SOUP SPICY KOREAN

INGREDIENTS

- 2 oz. mung bean noodles (glass noodles or cellophane)
- 1 c. cooked rib meat shred (from rich broth beef recipe)
- 2 tbsp. sesame oil
- 1 1/2 and a half to two tbsp. Korean red pepper flakes
- 1 tbsp. chopped garlic
- 4 c. Rich Beef Broth
- 1 c. water
- 2 c. chopped bok Choy
- 4 fresh sliced shitake mushrooms
- 2 scallions cut into 2 inches lengths
- For serving; Korean red pepper flakes
- For serving; Fish or soy sauce

DIRECTIONS

1. Soak the mung bean noodles for 20 to 30 minutes in hot water; rinse.
2. In a small skillet, heat red pepper flakes, sesame oil, and garlic until fragrant and light brown with garlic; combine with meat shredded; set aside.
3. Heat a large saucepan with beef broth and water. Add mushrooms, bok Choy, soaked mung bean noodles; cook until noodles are softened, and bok Choy are cooked around 3-4 minutes. To the soup, add scallions and marinated meat, and cook. Divide between bowls; for spicy food enthusiasts, serve with additional Korean red pepper flakes. Offer with fish or soy sauce, if the beef broth is unsalted.

NUTRITION

- Calories: 314
- Fat: 8g (5g sat)
- Protein: 22g
- Carb: 18g

- Sodium: 677mg
- Sugars: 1g
- Fiber: 1g

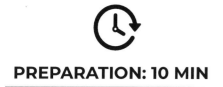
PREPARATION: 10 MIN

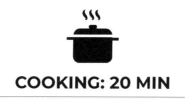
COOKING: 20 MIN

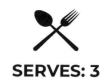
SERVES: 3

ASIAN-INSPIRED PORK CHOPS

INGREDIENTS

- 3 Pork chops, thinly-sliced center cut
- 2 tbsp Bragg Liquid Aminos/Sub. For soy sauce/or another favorite keto-friendly
- .5 tsp Garlic powder
- 1 pinch Salt
- .5 tsp Black pepper
- .5 tsp Ginger
- 2 tsp Minced garlic
- 1 tbsp Diced onions

DIRECTIONS

1. Mince the garlic and dice the onions. Toss everything into a zipper-type plastic bag. Shake the fixings.
2. Put the pork chops in a bag. Marinate two to 24 hours in the fridge, turning the bag from time to time.
3. Discard the marinade and drain the meat.
4. Grill them for 12-15 minutes using the medium temperature setting or until the desired doneness.

NUTRITION

- Calories: 106.1
- Net Carbohydrates: 2.7g
- Protein: 11.5g
- Fat Content: 5.5g

PREPARATION: 1 HOUR

COOKING: 7-9 HOURS

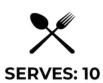
SERVES: 10

CROCKPOT PORK CHOPS

INGREDIENTS

- About 10 Pork chops (Family pack)
- 1 can Low-sodium/low-fat cream/mushroom/chicken celery, etc.
- .5 cup Ketchup

DIRECTIONS

1. Arrange the chops in the cooker. Add the ketchup and soup of choice.
2. Stir and close the lid. Place the timer on for seven to nine hours on the low setting.

NUTRITION

- Calories: 239.7
- Net Carbohydrates: 7.7g
- Protein: 21.8g
- Fat Content: 12.1g

PREPARATION: 10 MIN

COOKING: 35 MIN

SERVES: 4

HOT TEX-MEX PORK CASSEROLE

INGREDIENTS

- 2 tbsp Butter
- 1.5 lb Ground pork
- 3 tbsp Tex-Mex seasoning
- 2 tbsp Jalapenos
- .5 cupMonterey jack shredded cheese
- .5 cup Crushed tomatoes
- Serving & Garnish:
- 1 Scallion
- 1 cup Sour cream

DIRECTIONS

1. Warm the oven to reach 330° Fahrenheit.
2. Lightly spritz a baking tray using a cooking oil spray.
3. Add the butter to a skillet with the pork, and cook it for about eight minutes or until browned. Add the jalapenos, Tex-Mex, pepper, salt, and tomatoes. Simmer it for about five minutes.
4. Dump the fixings into the prepared dish and drizzle it with the cheese.
5. Set the timer for 20 minutes until its golden brown.
6. Garnish as desired.

NUTRITION

- Calories: 431
- Net Carbohydrates: 7.8g
- Protein: 43g

- Fat Content: 24g

PREPARATION: 1 HOUR

COOKING: 7-9 HOURS

SERVES: 4

MAPLE COUNTRY-STYLE PORK RIBS SLOW-COOKED

INGREDIENTS

- .25 tsp Ground allspice
- .25 tsp Ground cinnamon
- 2 lb. before cooked, Country-style pork ribs (will yield 16 oz. meat)
- .25 cup Onion
- .5 tsp Garlic powder
- 1 tbsp Maple-flavored syrup- no sugar
- 1 dash Black pepper
- .25 tsp Ground ginger
- 1 tbsp Low-sodium soy sauce

DIRECTIONS

1. Dice the onion and measure the rest of the components. Toss all of the fixings except for the ribs into a mixing container.
2. Pour the sauce over the ribs.
3. Pop it into a crockpot to cook with the lid 'on' using the low setting for seven to nine hours.

NUTRITION

- Calories: 188.4
- Net Carbohydrates: 2g
- Protein: 22.3g

- Fat Content: 9.4g

PREPARATION: 10 MIN

COOKING: 40 MIN

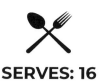
SERVES: 16

KOFTA KEBAB

INGREDIENTS

- 1 lb Ground lamb
- 1 lb 85% ground beef
- .5 cup Yellow onion
- 1 cup Fresh parsley
- 2 Garlic cloves
- Black pepper & salt
- Spices Used–1 tsp. Each:
- Ground nutmeg
- Sumac
- Ground green cardamom
- Ground allspice
- Also Needed: 16 wooden skewers

DIRECTIONS

1. Soak the skewers in water for at least one hour before it's time to grill.
2. Chop the onion, garlic, and parsley.
3. Toss all of the fixings into a large mixing container. Fold the spices into the meat mixture using your hands until it's thoroughly combined.
4. Portion the meat into ¼-cup portions and press them onto the skewer in a log shape.
5. Grill the kebabs until the internal temperature reaches 160° Fahrenheit, and it's nicely browned. Remove the kebabs from the grill, cover with foil, and wait for at least five minutes before serving.
6. Serve with grilled vegetables and our Tzatziki sauce for a delicious meal.

NUTRITION

- Calories: 145
- Net Carbohydrates: 1g
- Fat Content: 11g
- Protein: 10g

15. SEAFOODS

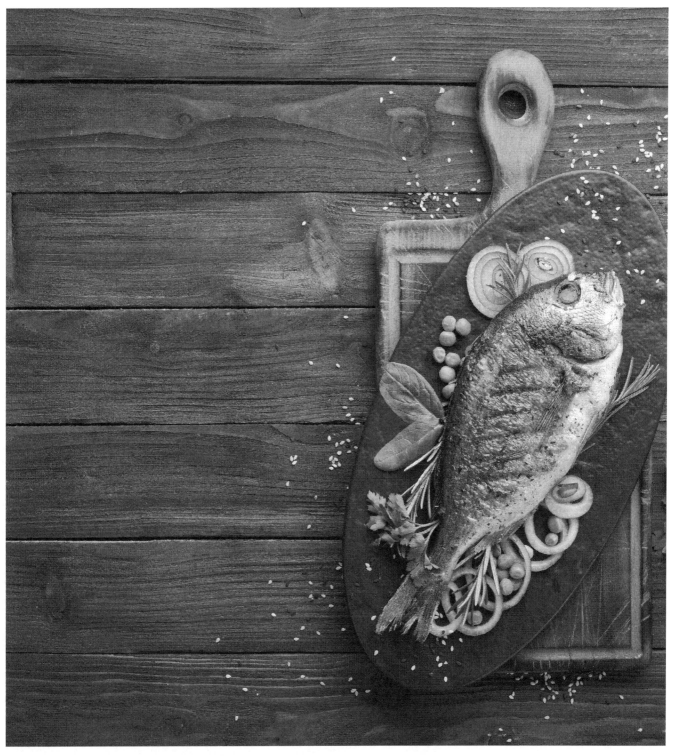

PREPARATION: 10 MIN

COOKING: 30 MIN

SERVES: 3

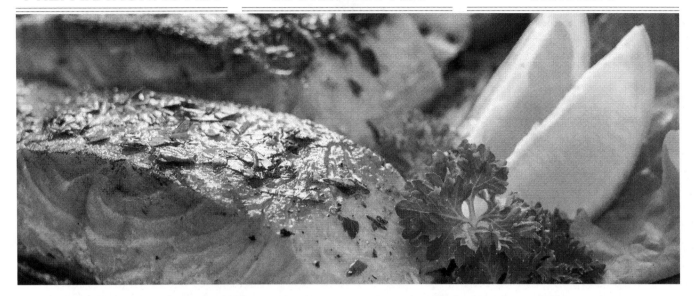

KETO BAKED SALMON WITH LEMON AND BUTTER

INGREDIENTS

- 1 pound salmon
- 1 lemon
- 3 oz. butter
- 1 tablespoon olive oil
- Ground black pepper and sea salt to taste

DIRECTIONS

1. Grease a large-sized baking dish with the olive oil and preheat your oven to 400°F.
2. Place the salmon on the baking dish, preferably skin-side down. Generously season with pepper and salt to taste.
3. Thinly slice the lemon and place the slices over the salmon. Cover the fish with ½ of the butter, preferably in very thin slices.
4. Bake until the salmon flakes easily with a fork and is opaque, for 25 to 30 minutes, on middle rack.
5. Now, over moderate heat in a small sauce pan; heat the remaining butter until it begins to bubble. Immediately remove the pan from heat; set aside and let cool a bit. Gently add in some of the freshly squeezed lemon juice.
6. Serve the cooked fish with some of the prepared lemon butter and enjoy.

NUTRITION

- Calories: 576
- Total Fat: 46g
- Saturated Fat: 22g
- Total Carbohydrates: 1.3g
- Dietary Fiber: 0.4g
- Sugars: 0.4g
- Protein: 31g

PREPARATION: 10 MIN

 COOKING: 5 MIN

 SERVES: 2

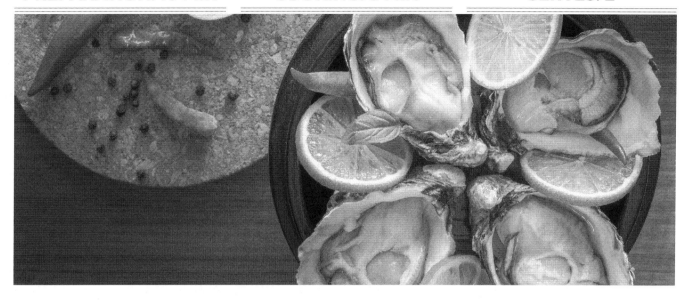

KETOGENIC SPICY OYSTER

INGREDIENTS

- 12 oysters shucked
- 1 tablespoon olive oil
- 7-8 basil leaves, fresh
- 1 tablespoon garlic chili paste
- 1/8 teaspoon salt

DIRECTIONS

1. Combine olive oil with garlic chili paste and salt in a medium size mixing bowl; mix well.
2. Add oysters into the prepared sauce; turning them several times until thoroughly coated.
3. Create a bed for the oysters to cook by spreading the basil leaves out on an oven-safe dish.
4. Transfer the oysters and sauce over the bed of basil leaves; spreading them in a single layer on the dish.
5. Turn on the broiler over high-heat.
6. Place the dish on top rack (approximately a few inches away from the broiler) and broil for a few minutes.
7. Once done; immediately remove them from the oven. Serve hot and enjoy.

NUTRITION

- Calories: 576
- Total Fat: 46g
- Saturated Fat: 22g
- Total Carbohydrates: 1.3g

- Dietary Fiber: 0.4g
- Sugars: 0.4g
- Protein: 31g

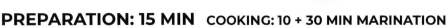
GARLIC LIME MAHI-MAHI

INGREDIENTS

- 4 Mahi-Mahi filets (approximately 1 to 1 ¼ pounds)
- Zest and juice of 1 large lime, fresh
- ¼ cup avocado oil
- 3 garlic cloves, minced
- 1/8 teaspoon each of ground black pepper and fine grain sea salt

DIRECTIONS

1. For Marinade: Thoroughly combine the entire ingredients (except the filets) together in a small-sized mixing bowl. Pour the mixture on top of filets in a large zip-lock bag or large shallow dish. Let marinate for 30 minutes, at room temperature.
2. Pour the marinade into a large sauté pan (preferably with a cover) and heat it over medium heat. Once hot; carefully add the filets into the hot pan; cover and cook the filets for a couple of minutes until cooked through.
3. Immediately remove the sauté pan from heat; set aside and let rest for 5 minutes, covered. Serve warm and enjoy.

NUTRITION

- Calories: 576
- Total Fat: 46g
- Saturated Fat: 22g
- Total Carbohydrates: 1.3g

- Dietary Fiber: 0.4g
- Sugars: 0.4g
- Protein: 31g

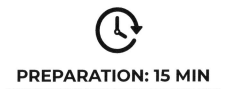

PREPARATION: 15 MIN

COOKING: 10 MIN

SERVES: 2

FISH AND LEEK SAUTÉ

INGREDIENTS

- 1 leek, chopped
- 2 trout fillets, diced (approximately 8 oz.)
- 1 tablespoon tamari soy sauce
- 1 teaspoon ginger, grated
- 1 tablespoon avocado oil
- Salt to taste

DIRECTIONS

1. Over moderate heat in a large skillet; heat the avocado oil until hot. Once done; add and sauté the chopped leek for a few minutes, until turn soften.
2. Immediately add the diced trout with grated ginger, tamari sauce and salt to taste.
3. Continue to sauté the trout until it's not translucent anymore and cooked through.
4. Serve immediately and enjoy.

NUTRITION

- Calories: 576
- Total Fat: 46g
- Saturated Fat: 22g
- Total Carbohydrates: 1.3g
- Dietary Fiber: 0.4g
- Sugars: 0.4g
- Protein: 31g

PREPARATION: 5 MIN

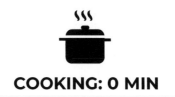
COOKING: 0 MIN

SERVES: 1

SMOKED SALMON SALAD

INGREDIENTS

- 2 oz. smoked salmon
- 1 lemon slice
- 4 olives
- 1 teaspoon pink peppercorns, crushed lightly
- A handful of arugula salad leaves, fresh

DIRECTIONS

1. Place the olives and salad leaves into a large plate or shallow bowl.
2. Arrange the smoked salmon over the salad.
3. Sprinkle the top of smoked salmon with lightly crushed pink peppercorns.
4. Garnish your salad with a lemon slice; serve immediately and enjoy.

NUTRITION

- Calories: 149
- Total Fat: 5.2g
- Saturated Fat: 1.4g
- Total Carbohydrates: 4g
- Dietary Fiber: 1.7g
- Sugars: 3.4g
- Protein: 11g

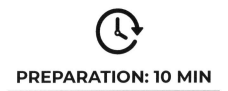

PREPARATION: 10 MIN

COOKING: 30 MIN

SERVES: 2

KETO BAKED SALMON WITH PESTO

INGREDIENTS

- 1 oz. green pesto
- ½ pound salmon
- Pepper and salt to taste
- For Green sauce:
- ¼ cup Greek yogurt
- 1 oz. green pesto
- ¼ teaspoon garlic
- Pepper and salt to taste

DIRECTIONS

1. Preheat your oven to 400°F.
2. Arrange the salmon in a well-greased baking dish, preferably skin-side down. Spread the pesto over the salmon and then, sprinkle with pepper and salt to taste.
3. Bake in the preheated oven until the salmon flakes easily with a fork, for 25 to 30 minutes.
4. In the meantime, stir the entire sauce ingredients together in a large bowl. Serve the cooked fish with some of the prepared sauce and enjoy.

NUTRITION

- Calories: 274
- Total Fat: 21g
- Saturated Fat: 3.9g
- Total Carbohydrates: 2.9g

- Dietary Fiber: 0.6g
- Sugars: 1.7g
- Protein: 26g

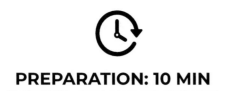
PREPARATION: 10 MIN

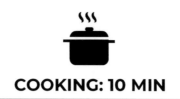
COOKING: 10 MIN

SERVES: 2

ROASTED SALMON WITH PARMESAN DILL CRUST

INGREDIENTS

- ½ pound salmon; cut into pieces
- 1 tablespoon dill weed
- ¼ cup cottage cheese
- 1 tablespoon olive oil
- ¼ cup parmesan cheese, grated

DIRECTIONS

1. Preheat your oven to 450°F.
2. Combine cottage cheese with parmesan cheese, olive oil and dill in a large-sized mixing bowl; mix well.
3. Line a large-sized baking sheet with aluminum foil and then, arrange the salmon pieces on it.
4. Smear ½ of the cottage cheese mix over the salmon.
5. Roast in the preheated oven until the fish flakes easily and crust is brown, for 10 minutes.
6. Serve the cooked fish with the remaining prepared sauce and enjoy.

NUTRITION

- Calories: 352
- Total Fat: 22g
- Saturated Fat: 6.6g
- Total Carbohydrates: 5.7g
- Dietary Fiber: 1.5g
- Sugars: 0.5g
- Protein: 33g

PREPARATION: 15 MIN

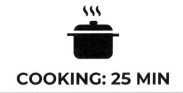

COOKING: 25 MIN

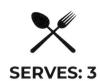

SERVES: 3

KETO FRIED SALMON WITH BROCCOLI AND CHEESE

INGREDIENTS

- ¾ pound salmon; cut into pieces
- 3 tablespoons butter
- ½ pound broccoli; cut into small florets
- 2 oz. cheddar cheese, grated
- Pepper and salt to taste
- 1 lime

DIRECTIONS

1. Preheat your oven using the broiler settings, to 400°F.
2. Let the broccoli florets to simmer for a couple of minutes, preferably in lightly salted water. Ensure that the broccoli maintains its delicate color and chewy texture; drain well.
3. Now arrange the broccoli in a baking dish, preferably well-greased. Add butter and pepper to taste.
4. Sprinkle with cheese and bake in the preheated oven until the cheese turns golden in color, for 15 to 20 minutes.
5. Now, over moderate heat in a large saucepan; heat the butter until completely melted and fry the salmon pieces for a couple of minutes per side. Serve the pan-fried salmon with baked broccoli and enjoy.

NUTRITION

- Calories: 392
- Total Fat: 25g
- Saturated Fat: 11.8g
- Total Carbohydrates: 5.8g
- Dietary Fiber: 3.4g
- Sugars: 1.4g
- Protein: 31g

PREPARATION: 15 MIN

COOKING: 15 MIN

SERVES: 2

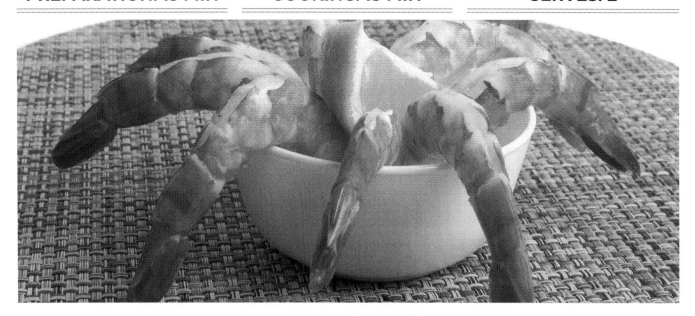

TANGY SHRIMP

INGREDIENTS

- 3garlic cloves
- .25 cup olive oil
- .5lb. Jumbo shrimp
- 1 lemon
- Cayenne pepper

DIRECTIONS

1. Sauté the garlic and cayenne with the olive oil. Peel and devein the shrimp. Cook within 2 to 3 minutes per side. Put pepper, salt, and lemon wedges. Use the rest of the garlic oil for a dipping sauce. Serve.

NUTRITION

- Net Carbohydrates: 3grams
- Protein: 23grams
- Total Fats: 27grams

- Calories: 335

PREPARATION: 30 MIN

COOKING: 40 MIN

SERVES: 5 (4 PIECES EACH)

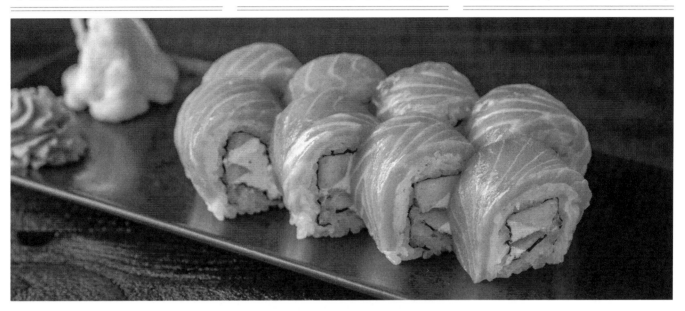

SALMON SUSHI ROLLS

INGREDIENTS

- 4 oz. smoked salmon
- ¼ red bell pepper, cut into matchstick pieces
- ½ cucumber, cut into matchstick pieces
- ½ avocado
- 20 seaweed sheets
- ½ cup Water

DIRECTIONS

1. Cut the salmon and avocado the same way that you cut the red pepper and cucumber.
2. Place seaweed snacks on a cutting board.
3. Put a cup of water nearby. Wet your fingers with water and wet one edge of each seaweed sheet.
4. Put one piece of salmon, pepper, cucumber, and avocado on each seaweed snack and roll them up.

NUTRITION

- Calories: 320
- Fat: 20grams
- Net Carbs: 8grams

- Protein: 24grams

PREPARATION: 35 MIN

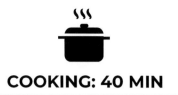
COOKING: 40 MIN

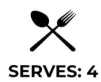
SERVES: 4

SHRIMP LETTUCE WRAPS WITH BUFFALO SAUCE

INGREDIENTS

- 1 egg, beaten
- 3 tablespoons butter
- 16 oz. shrimp, peeled, deveined, with tails removed
- ¾ cup almond flour
- ¼ cup hot sauce (like Frank's)
- 1 teaspoon extra-virgin olive oil
- Kosher salt
- Black pepper
- Garlic
- 1 head romaine lettuce, leaves parted, for serving
- ½ red onion, chopped
- Celery, finely sliced
- ½ blue cheese, cut into pieces

DIRECTIONS

1. To make the Buffalo sauce, melt the butter in a saucepan, add the garlic and cook this mixture for 1 minute. Pour hot sauce into the saucepan and whisk to combine.
2. Set aside.
3. In one bowl, crack one egg, add salt and pepper and mix. In another bowl, put the almond flour, add salt and pepper and also combine.
4. Dip each shrimp into the egg mixture first and then into the almond one.
5. Take a large frying pan. Heat the oil and cook your shrimp for about 2 minutes per side.
6. Add Buffalo sauce.
7. Serve in lettuce leaves. Top your shrimp with red onion, blue cheese, and celery.

NUTRITION

- Calories: 606
- Fat: 54grams
- Net Carbs: 8grams

- Protein: 33grams

SHRIMP SCAMPI WITH GARLIC

INGREDIENTS

- 1 pound shrimp
- 3 tablespoons olive oil
- 1 bulb shallot, sliced
- 4 garlic cloves minced
- ½ cup Pinot Grigio
- 4 tablespoons salted butter
- 1 tablespoon lemon juice
- ½ teaspoon of sea salt
- ¼ teaspoon black pepper
- ¼ teaspoon red pepper flakes
- ¼ cup parsley, chopped

DIRECTIONS

1. Pour the olive oil into the previously heated frying pan. Add the garlic and shallots and fry for about 2 minutes.
2. Combine the Pinot Grigio, salted butter, and lemon juice. Pour this mix into the pan and cook for 5 minutes.
3. Put the parsley, black pepper, red pepper flakes, and sea salt into the pan and whisk well.
4. Add the shrimp and fry until they are pink (about 3 minutes).

NUTRITION

- Calories: 344
- Fat: 7grams
- Net Carbs: 7grams

- Protein: 32grams

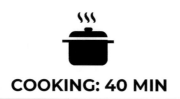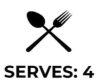
BAKED TILAPIA

INGREDIENTS

- 4 tilapia fillets
- 1 lemon zest
- 2 tablespoons fresh lemon juice
- 1 tablespoon garlic, minced
- ¼ cup butter, melted
- 2 tablespoons fresh parsley, chopped
- Pepper
- Salt

DIRECTIONS

1. Preheat the oven to 4250 F.
2. In a small bowl, mix together butter, lemon zest, lemon juice, and garlic and set aside.
3. Season fish fillets with pepper and salt.
4. Place fish fillets onto the baking dish. Pour butter mixture over fish fillets.
5. Bake fish in a preheated oven for 10-12 minutes.
6. Garnish with parsley and serve.

NUTRITION

- Calories: 247
- Fat: 13.6grams
- Net Carbs: 1gram
- Protein: 32.4grams

16. POULTRY

PREPARATION: 10 MIN

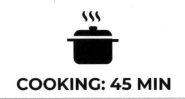

COOKING: 45 MIN

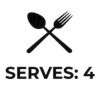

SERVES: 4

BROCCOLI CHEDDAR CHICKEN FROM CRACKER BARREL

INGREDIENTS

- ½ tsp. salt
- 1 cup of milk
- ½ tsp. paprika
- 8 oz. frozen chopped broccoli
- ½ tsp. pepper
- 4 chicken breast–boneless and skinless
- 1 can of cheddar cheese soup
- 1 ½ cups of crushed Ritz crackers
- 6 oz. cheddar cheese, shredded

DIRECTIONS

1. Start by preheating the oven. Set the oven temperature at 350 degrees Fahrenheit. Grease a casserole dish slightly.
2. Mix salt and pepper. Use it to season the chicken and keep the chicken aside in a prepared dish.
3. Use a medium-sized bowl, add the milk, paprika, soup, and cheddar cheese. Mix them thoroughly.
4. On the chicken, pour about half of the cream mixture and a dash of the broccoli pieces.
5. Use the Ritz cracker pieces and cheese mixture as the topping.
6. Bake it for 45 minutes in the preheated oven.

Note: For a crunchy topping, mixer the cracker crumbs with melted butter of one or two tbsp. Sprinkle this over the top.

NUTRITION

- Calories: 690
- Protein: 40g
- Carbs: 20g
- Fats: 44g
- Fiber: 5g

PREPARATION: 10 MIN

COOKING: 40 MIN

SERVES: 6

CHICKEN BAKE FROM COSTCO

INGREDIENTS

- ½ cup of parmesan
- 3 cups of mozzarella cheese
- 1 cup of bacon crisps
- 2 cups of cooked chicken
- 1 ½ lb. pizza dough
- Flour
- 1 cup of Ranch dressing

DIRECTIONS

1. Divide the dough into six parts.
2. Roll them into rectangular shapes. Leaving about an inch on all the sides, apply the ranch on the rolled dough. Top the dough with bacon and chicken
3. Place a handful of mozzarella cheese. Roll the dough slowly. Use a baking sheet and grease it with oil. Place the rolls one by one carefully on the baking sheet greased with oil.
4. On the outside of the rolls, apply the ranch in a small quantity using a brush.
5. Set a timer to bake at 415 degrees Fahrenheit (17-20 min.). When the time is over, transfer the pan to the stovetop.
6. Sprinkle them using a portion of the parmesan cheese on the rolls. Again, bake the rolls in the oven. Do not bake for more than five minutes. Keep in mind that you need to get golden brown rolls.
7. Serve immediately—while the cheese is in a melted state.

Note: The pizza dough should be purchased or made before you start making the recipe. If you are using full-portion pizza dough, double the recipe, or save the rest of the dough in the refrigerator for another time.

NUTRITION

- Calories: 571
- Protein: 30g
- Carbs: 19g
- Fats: 41g

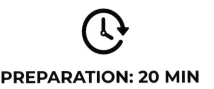
PREPARATION: 20 MIN

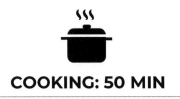
COOKING: 50 MIN

SERVES: 6

CHICKEN CASSEROLE FROM CRACKER BARREL

INGREDIENTS

- The Cornbread:
- ⅓ cup of flour, all-purpose
- 1 ½ tsp. baking powder
- 1 cup yellow cornmeal
- ½ tsp. salt
- 1 tbsp. sugar
- ¾ cup of buttermilk
- 1 egg
- ½ tsp. baking soda
- ½ cup of butter, melted
- The Filling:
- 2 ½ cups of chicken breast
- ¼ cup of yellow onion
- ½ cup celery
- 1 ¾ cups of chicken broth
- 2 tbsp. butter
- oz. can of cream of chicken soup
- 1 tsp. salt
- ¼ tsp. pepper

DIRECTIONS

1. Do the Prep: Chop the chicken into bite-sized pieces. Thinly slice the celery and chop the onion.
2. For Cornbread: In a mixing bowl, whisk the yellow cornmeal, all-purpose flour, egg, buttermilk, baking soda, vegetable oil, sugar, salt, and baking powder. Combine thoroughly to form a smooth mixture.
3. Grease an eight-inch square baking pan. Pour the batter into it. At 375 degrees Fahrenheit, bake in the oven. The time should be around 20-25 minutes. Or, bake till the batter turns golden brown. When it is finished, transfer the bread to the countertop and let it cool.
4. When the cornbread is completely cool, you need to crumble all of it. Then, take three cups of the cornbread crumbles and toss them into a mixing container. Mix in the melted butter to the crumbles. Mix thoroughly and set it aside.
5. For Chicken Filling: You need a pan of medium size. Heat in the flame of medium to a high level. Add the butter into it, and heat it. Sauté the chopped celery and onions in this pan until they are translucent.
6. Now to the pan, add the cream of chicken soup, pepper, salt, and chicken broth. Keep stirring. The ingredients should be thoroughly blended. Stir till the soup is completely dissolved.
7. Add the cooked chicken into this pan. Continue stirring until everything blends using a low simmer. Keep cooking for another five minutes. After that, take the pan off from the stove.
8. Use a casserole dish or four individual casserole dishes. Butter the container/dishes, and place the chicken filling into them.
9. Generously scatter the cornbread crumbles over the chicken mixture. (Never stir the chicken filling. All you need to do is to form a crust on that filling.)
10. Preheat an oven at 350 degrees Fahrenheit. Set a timer and bake it for about thirty-five to 35-40 minutes. This ensures the crumbles turn golden yellow. Place the baking dish into the oven.
11. Remove when done. Serve when hot.

Note: Substitute cream of mushroom or potato soup instead of the cream of chicken soup if desired.

NUTRITION

- Calories: 457
- Protein: 45g
- Carbs: 6g
- Fat: 27g
- Fiber: 2g

PREPARATION: 2H

COOKING: 18H 15 MIN

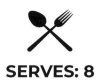
SERVES: 8

CHIPOTLE CHICKEN

INGREDIENTS

- 1 oz. each:
- Dried ancho chili pepper
- Dried chipotle chili pepper
- 4garlic cloves
- ½ red onion
- 2 tbsp. of olive oil
- ½ cup of water
- 1 tsp. each:
- Black pepper (freshly ground)
- Dried oregano
- Ground cumin
- lb. of chicken thighs (boneless & skinless)
- 2 tsp. of sea salt

DIRECTIONS

1. Grab a bowl and in it, add the two types of Chile peppers. Mix in the water. Allow the peppers to become softened for about 12 hours. After that, remove the peppers and eliminate the seeds.
2. Use the bowl of a blender and, in it, add red onion, Chile peppers, cumin, sea salt, garlic, black pepper, and oregano. Blend everything until you get a coarse paste. Add the olive oil and blend again until it reaches a smooth mixture.
3. Use a meat mallet to smash the chicken thighs. Trim away any excess skin. Take a zipper-type plastic bag and add the chicken and the marinade. Shake the bag to ensure all the chicken pieces have coated evenly with the marinade. Leave the bag to marinate for eight hours in the fridge.
4. Put the bottom and top plates on your outdoor grill and preheat using the med-high temperature setting.
5. Discard the marinade and transfer the chicken onto the heated grill.
6. Cook the chicken for about ten minutes. The juices will run clear by this time, and there will be no pinkish region in the center. Cut the chicken into strips and serve.

NUTRITION

- Calories: 293
- Protein: 24.9g
- Carbs: 5.8g
- Fats: 18.7g
- Fibre: 2.1g

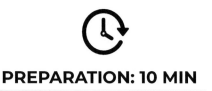

PREPARATION: 10 MIN

COOKING: 45 MIN

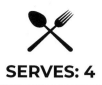

SERVES: 4

CHICKEN LETTUCE WRAPS FROM PF CHANG'S

INGREDIENTS

- For the Marinade:
- 2 tsp. soy sauce
- 2 tbsp. of sherry/red wine
- 2 tsp. cornstarch
- 2 tsp. water
- Filling Ingredients for Lettuce Wraps:
- 1 tsp. ginger
- ½ cup minced shiitake mushrooms
- 8 oz. minced water chestnuts
- 8 oz. minced bamboo shoots
- 1 ½ lb. chicken breasts–boneless & skinless
- 5 tbsp. vegetable/peanut oil
- ½ cup minced garlic
- 6 oz. Chinese cellophane noodles
- ½ cup green onions
- Cooking Sauce:
- 1 tsp. sugar
- 2 tbsp. water
- 1 tbsp. soy sauce
- 1 tsp. sesame oil
- 2 tbsp. oyster sauce
- 1 tbsp. Hoisin sauce
- 1 tbsp. sherry wine or red wine
- 2 tsp. cornstarch
- 1 head of iceberg lettuce-washed and left whole after taken off the head

DIRECTIONS

1. Mince the veggies as desired.
2. Thoroughly mix the ingredients listed for the cooking sauce. Set aside for now.
3. In another mixing container, thoroughly mix the ingredients for the marinade. Add the chicken to this. Stir well and coat the chicken evenly.
4. Mix in one teaspoon of oil and let it rest for 15 minutes. On a medium-high flame, heat a large wok or a large skillet. While it gets heated, chop the chicken into small pieces. To the skillet or wok, add three tablespoons of oil. Stir fry the chicken in it for three to four minutes. Dump the mixture into a holding container, and place it to the side.
5. Add two tablespoons of oil to the same pan.
6. Stir fry the ginger, garlic, and onion, for a minute in the pan. Add the bamboo shoots, water chestnuts, and mushrooms. Toss to fry for two more minutes. Mix in the chicken to the pan, followed by the cooking sauce you have previously mixed. Cook until it is hot and thickened.
7. Cook the cellophane noodles, and break them apart. In the serving dish, cover the bottom with these noodles. Pour the chicken mixture on top of it. Serve with lettuce leaves.

Note: If you feel like making ahead of time, you can make the fillings and pop them into the fridge for two days. When you want to use them, all you need to do is microwave or heat them in a large skillet. If you have any leftovers, store them in the fridge for up to five days. Unfortunately, the leftover filling with lettuce will turn soggy, and this cannot be refrigerated.

NUTRITION

- Calories: 269
- Carbs: 8g
- Protein: 33g
- Fat: 11g
- Fiber: 2g

PREPARATION: 10 MIN

COOKING: 30 MIN

SERVES: 5

CHICKEN PICCATA FROM OLIVE GARDEN

INGREDIENTS

- 4 chicken breasts
- 1 small onion
- ¼ cup capers
- 10 sun-dried tomatoes
- 1 tbsp. garlic
- 1 ½ cups chicken broth
- 3 tbsp. butter
- ⅓ cup heavy cream
- ½ of 1 lemon, juiced– about 2 tbsp.
- Black pepper & salt as desired
- For Frying: 4 tbsp. olive oil

DIRECTIONS

1. Pound the chicken using a mallet until it's about a ¼-inch thickness and dust with salt and pepper.
2. Cook using the med-high temperature setting until golden and thoroughly cooked (approx. 5-8 min. per side.) Transfer the chicken to a holding container and set it to the side.
3. Slice the tomatoes into strips and mince the garlic. Use the same skillet to add the garlic, sun-dried tomatoes, and onions. Sauté until lightly browned (one to two minutes).
4. Rinse and drain the capers.
5. Whisk in the capers with the chicken broth and lemon juice. Take a minute to remove the tasty bits from the pan using a wooden spoon. Simmer the sauce using the med-low temperature setting to reduce in size by about half the volume (10-15 min.).
6. Once the sauce has thickened, remove the pan to a cool burner. Whisk in the butter. Once it's melted, mix in the cream and thoroughly warm the fixings (½ minute).
7. It's time to serve after you cover the breasts in the delicious sauce.

Notes: Use one to two tablespoons of the sun-dried tomato oil to replace part of the olive oil for a change of pace.

NUTRITION

- Calories: 451
- Protein: 40g
- Carbs: 6g
- Fat: 29g
- Fiber: 1g

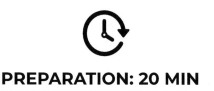
PREPARATION: 20 MIN

COOKING: 50 MIN

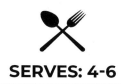
SERVES: 4-6

EASY MALIBU CHICKEN FROM SIZZLER STEAK HOUSE

INGREDIENTS

- 4 breasts of chicken (6 oz. each)
- Salt & black pepper
- The Dipping Sauce:
- 3 tbsp. Dijon/ yellow mustard/combo if desired
- ½ cup mayonnaise
- 1-2 tbsp. keto-friendly powdered sugar
- The Crumb Topping:
- ¾ cup/36g crushed pork rinds or panko crumbs
- ¾ cup /60g of grated parmesan cheese
- 2 tsp. granulated garlic
- ⅛ tsp. pepper
- 1 tsp. granulated onion
- ¼ tsp. salt
- The Topping:
- 8 or a total of 6 oz, thinly sliced deli ham
- 4 slices or a total of 4 oz Swiss cheese
- Also Needed: 9 by 13-inch baking dish, glass is preferred

DIRECTIONS

1. Warm the oven at 350 degrees Fahrenheit. Arrange the oven rack in the center-most position. Finely crush the pork rinds. You can use a rolling pin and crush them in a plastic bag or use a food processor.
2. Prepare the chicken by patting it dry. Sprinkle it using a portion of pepper and salt.
3. Mix the mustard, sweetener, and mayo in a mixing container.
4. Add ¼ cup of the mustard mixture to the plate with the chicken, saving the rest as the dipping sauce. Roll the chicken in the mix.
5. Note: You can also place the chicken in a bowl and mix it with the mustard mix and marinate it for up to one day. The chicken can also be cooked right away after you marinate it for ½ hour or so.
6. Combine the seasonings with the crushed pork rinds and parmesan. Sprinkle half of the crumb mixture into the baking container.
7. Add the chicken and the remainder of the crumb mixture over the chicken.
8. Bake it until the chicken is thoroughly cooked (30-40 min.).
9. Transfer the pan to the stovetop on a cool burner and add the ham and cheese. Pop the dish back into the oven. Serve after the cheese has melted.

NUTRITION

- Calories: 696
- Protein: 46g
- Carbs: 4g
- Fat: 55g

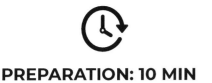
PREPARATION: 10 MIN

COOKING: 35 MIN

SERVES: 4

GARLIC ROSEMARY CHICKEN FROM OLIVE GARDEN

INGREDIENTS

- 2 tbsp olive oil
- 3 cups baby spinach
- 2 cup mushrooms
- ½ tsp. of kosher salt
- 3 tbsp. of fresh rosemary
- 1 cup of chicken broth**
- 2 cloves of garlic
- 8 oz chicken breast
- ¼ tsp black pepper
- ¼ cup dry white wine

DIRECTIONS

1. Do the prep. Thinly slice the mushrooms. Mince the rosemary and garlic. Trim the chicken to remove all bones and fatty skin.
2. Pour one (1) tablespoon of olive oil in a big skillet and warm it using a moderate flame. After the oil becomes hot, toss in the mushrooms and garlic. Sauté and brown them for about eight minutes and remove.
3. In the remaining oil, add the chicken breasts, pepper, rosemary, and salt to season. Prepare it for eight minutes per side until the golden brown color is seen and then set aside.
4. Keep the flame at medium, add the mushrooms back to the skillet and add the chicken broth and wine. Simmer for five minutes to reduce the broth and add the spinach leaves. Cook thoroughly until the leaves get wilted.
5. Shift the chicken pieces to the serving plate. Top with spinach leaves and mushroom to serve.

Notes: Watch out for your health and use low-sodium chicken broth.

NUTRITION

- Calories: 336
- Carb: 4g
- Protein: 48g
- Fat: 13g
- Fiber: 1g

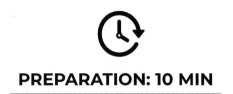

PREPARATION: 10 MIN

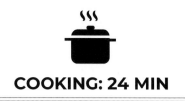

COOKING: 24 MIN

SERVES: 4

INSTANT POT CHICKEN FROM GENERAL TSO'S

INGREDIENTS

- For the Sauce:
- 1 tsp. sesame oil
- 2 tbsp no sugar added ketchup
- ½ tsp. ginger
- 5 tbsp. less-sodium soy sauce (gluten-free option - choose tamari)
- 1 tsp. chili paste
- 1 tsp. granular sweetener
- 3 garlic cloves
- For the Chicken:
- ¼ tsp. each of pepper and salt
- 1 ½ lb. chicken thigh meat- boneless
- 2 egg whites
- 2 tbsp coconut oil
- ½ tsp. xanthan gum
- ½ cup chicken broth
- ½ cup almond flour
- Optional: Green onion and sesame seeds–for garnishing

DIRECTIONS

1. Mince the ginger and garlic. In a bowl, mix the ingredients that are mentioned to make the sauce. Whisk them thoroughly and set aside.
2. Dice the chicken into small-sized pieces. Use pepper and salt for seasoning.
3. In two different bowls, place the egg whites and almond flour—separately. Rummage each chicken piece into the egg white first. Then coat with almond flour.
4. Use the sauté function to warm the coconut oil in an Instant pot.
5. Trim and add the chicken to it, and sauté it. If you are not able to do it in a single batch, do in multiple batches.
6. Deglaze the pot's bottom with the broth now. If small pieces are sticking at the bottom, get all of them with a spoon. Cover with the lid using the manual setting on the high mode, set for four minutes.
7. Release the pressure quickly and carefully. Using the back of the spoon is the right choice.
8. Thicken the sauce by whisking it with the xanthan gum. Cauliflower rice might be the perfect accompaniment for this recipe and keto-friendly too. You can garnish with green onion and sesame seeds if you prefer.

Note: In case you don't have an Instant Pot, try this in a slow cooker. For this, coat the chicken and brown it in a skillet. Add it to the slow cooker. Prepare the sauce and pour it over the chicken, followed by the broth. Leave the cooker covered in the low setting for four hours.

NUTRITION

- Calories: 427
- Protein: 35g
- Carbs: 7g
- Fats: 30g
- Fiber: 2g

17. VEGETABLES

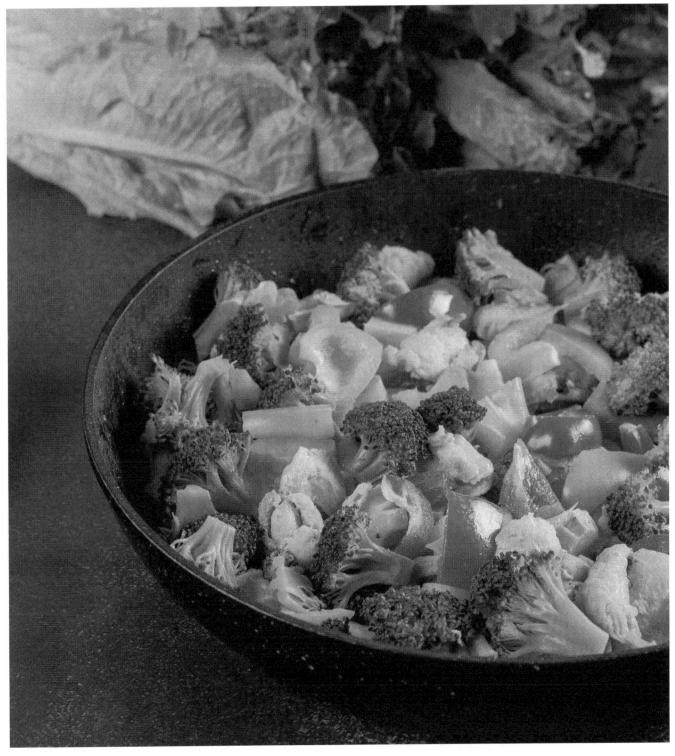

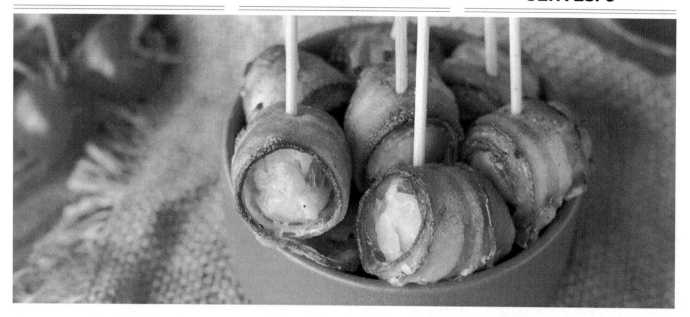

BRUSSELS SPROUTS WITH BACON

INGREDIENTS

- 16 oz. Bacon
- 16 oz. Brussels sprouts
- Black pepper

DIRECTIONS

1. Warm the oven to reach 400° Fahrenheit.
2. Slice the bacon into small lengthwise pieces. Put the sprouts and bacon with pepper.
3. Bake within 35 to 40 minutes. Serve.

NUTRITION

- Carbohydrates: 3.9grams
- Protein: 7.9grams
- Total Fats: 6.9grams
- Calories: 113

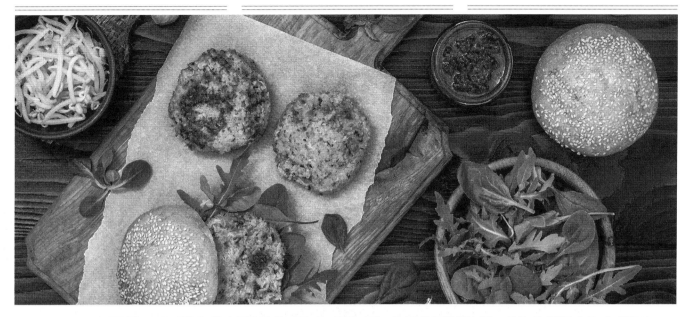

MIXED VEGETABLE PATTIES-INSTANT POT

INGREDIENTS

- 1 cup cauliflower florets
- 1 bag vegetables
- 1.5 cups Water
- 1 cup Flax meal
- 2 tbsp. Olive oil

DIRECTIONS

1. Steam the veggies to the steamer basket within 4 to 5 minutes. Mash in the flax meal. Shape into 4 patties. Cook the patties within 3 minutes per side. Serve.

NUTRITION

- Net Carbohydrates: 3grams
- Protein: 4grams
- Total Fats: 10grams

- Calories: 220

PREPARATION: 21 MIN

COOKING: 10 MIN

SERVES: 4

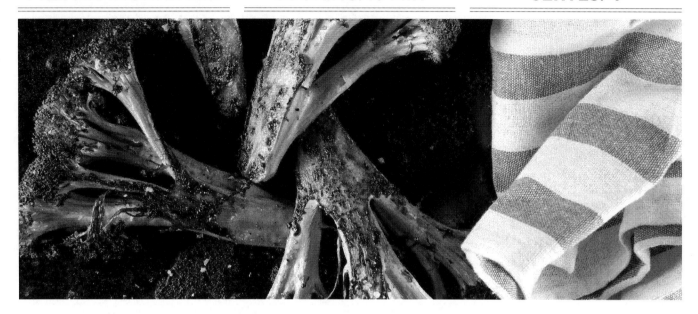

EASY ROASTED BROCCOLI

INGREDIENTS

- 1 pound frozen broccoli, cut into florets
- 3 teaspoons olive oil
- Sea salt, to taste

DIRECTIONS

1. Place broccoli florets on a baking sheet greased with oil and put it in the oven (preheated to 400°F). Sprinkle the olive oil over the florets.
2. Cook for 12 minutes. Whisk well and bake for an additional 7 minutes.

NUTRITION

- Calories: 58
- Fat: 3grams
- Net Carbs: 8grams
- Protein: 3grams

PREPARATION: 5 MIN

COOKING: 7 MIN

SERVES: 1

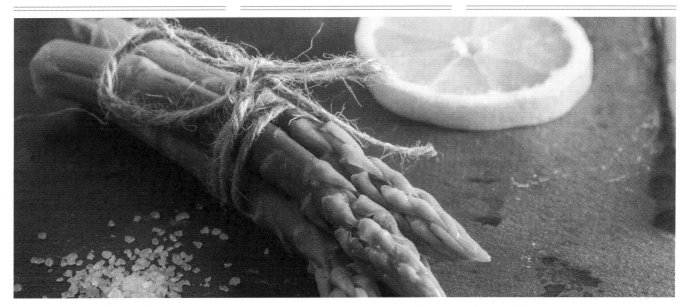

BOILED ASPARAGUS WITH SLICED LEMON

INGREDIENTS

- 10 large beans asparagus
- 3 Tbsp. avocado oil
- ¼ Tbsp. lemon juice
- 2-3 pieces lemon
- ¼ cup water
- ½ tsp. salt

DIRECTIONS

1. Place the asparagus in a pot of water. Boil for about 5-7 minutes.
2. Take the asparagus out of the pot. Sprinkle with lemon juice, avocado oil, and salt. Serve with the pieces of lemon.

NUTRITION

- Carbohydrates: 10.7g
- Fat: 43g
- Protein: 4.7g

- Calories: 447

PREPARATION: 10 MIN

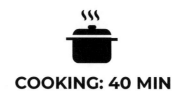

COOKING: 40 MIN

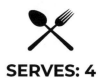

SERVES: 4

ROASTED CABBAGE WITH BACON

INGREDIENTS

- ½ head cabbage, quartered
- 8 slices bacon, cut into thick pieces
- ¼ cup Parmesan cheese, grated
- 1 tsp. garlic powder
- Salt and pepper, to taste
- 1 pinch parsley, chopped

DIRECTIONS

1. Lightly sprinkle the cabbage wedges with the garlic powder and parmesan cheese. Wrap 2 pieces of bacon around each cabbage wedge.
2. Place your wrapped cabbage wedges on the baking sheet and put into the oven preheated to 350°F oven. Bake for 35-40 minutes. Top with parsley.

NUTRITION

- Carbohydrates: 7g
- Fat: 19g
- Protein: 9g
- Calories: 236

PREPARATION: 10 MIN

COOKING: 40 MIN

SERVES: 4

LOADED CAULIFLOWER

INGREDIENTS

- 1 1/4 pound cauliflower head, cut into florets
- 6 green onion, chopped into the green and white parts
- 2 tablespoons butter
- 3 minced garlic cloves
- 2 oz. cream cheese
- 1/2 tablespoon sea salt
- 1/4 tablespoon black pepper
- 1/5 of a tablespoon ranch seasoning Mix, optional
- 3/4 c. organic heavy whipping cream
- 2 c. cheddar cheese, grated
- 4 sugar-free slices bacon
- Olive oil for cauliflower roasting
- Lumps of sour cream

DIRECTIONS

1. Heat the oven to a stage of 425 degrees.
2. Toss ~2 Tbsp. of olive oil with the cauliflower, then add it to a baking dish. For 25 minutes, roast the cauliflower on a baking dish. The cauliflower is going to be tender and certain sections may be brown.
3. Generate the cheese sauce when roasting the cauliflower: apply the sugar, the white pieces of the green onions, and the garlic cloves to a medium-hot skillet. Sauté (~3 minutes) until the onions are translucent.
4. Apply the onions, garlic, and butter to the pan with heavy cream, cream cheese, cinnamon, ranch seasoning (if you are using it), and pepper. Switch the heat down to mild and cook until the cream cheese is melted. To finish the cheese sauce, stir in 1.5 cups of cheddar cheese.
5. The cheese sauce and the roasted cauliflower are combined and then applied to a baking dish. Cover it with the leftover cheddar cheese and roast for an extra 20 minutes, or until the cauliflower is soft.
6. Top the fried cauliflower, the green pieces of the green onions, and the crumbled bacon with some globs of sour cream.

NUTRITION

- Calories: 315
- Fat: 28g (17g sat)
- Protein: 11g
- Carb: 5g
- Sodium: 587mg
- Sugars: 2g
- Fiber: 1g

PREPARATION: 5 MIN

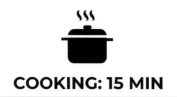
COOKING: 15 MIN

SERVES: 2

ZUCCHINI CAULIFLOWER FRITTERS

INGREDIENTS

- ¼ head of cauliflower, chopped (roughly 1 ½ cups)
- 1 tablespoon coconut oil
- 1/8 cup coconut flour
- 1 medium zucchini; grated
- Black pepper and sea salt to taste

DIRECTIONS

1. Steam the cauliflower until just fork tender, for 3 to 5 minutes. Add cauliflower to your food processor and process on high power until broken down into very small chunks (ensure it's not mashed).
2. Squeeze the moisture as much as possible from the grated veggies using a nut milk bag or dishtowel.
3. Transfer to a large bowl along with the grated zucchini and add flour coconut flour followed by pepper, salt and any seasonings you desire; combine well. Make 4 small-sized patties from the mixture.
4. Now, over moderate heat in a large pan; heat 1 tablespoon of coconut oil. Work in batches and cook the fritters for 2 to 3 minutes per side. The cooked fritters can be served with some dipping sauce of your choice on side.

NUTRITION

- Calories: 112
- Total Fat: 8g
- Saturated Fat: 5.8g
- Total Carbohydrates: 5.6g
- Dietary Fiber: 2.2g
- Sugars: 2g
- Protein: 2.1g

PREPARATION: 5 MIN

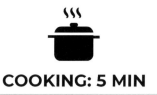

COOKING: 5 MIN

SERVES: 4

EGGLESS SALAD

INGREDIENTS

- 1 stalk celery, chopped
- Vegan mayonnaise, as required
- 1 pound extra firm tofu
- 2 tablespoons onions, minced
- Pepper and salt to taste

DIRECTIONS

1. Mash the tofu into a chunky texture, just like an egg salad.
2. Add mayonnaise until you get your desired consistency.
3. Add in the leftover ingredients; stir well.
4. Serve on keto pitas or keto bread, with vegetables and enjoy.

NUTRITION

- Calories: 117
- Total Fat: 7.8g
- Saturated Fat: 1.3g
- Total Carbohydrates: 2.8g
- Dietary Fiber: 1.5g
- Sugars: 1.4g
- Protein: 16g

PREPARATION: 5 MIN

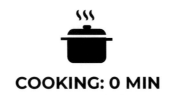
COOKING: 0 MIN

SERVES: 6

MOUTH-WATERING GUACAMOLE

INGREDIENTS

- 3 avocados, pitted
- ¼ cup cilantro, freshly chopped, plus more for garnish
- Juice of 2 limes
- ½ teaspoon kosher salt
- 1 small jalapeño, minced
- ½ small white onion, finely chopped

DIRECTIONS

1. Combine avocados with cilantro, lime juice, jalapeño, onion and salt in a large-sized mixing bowl; mix well.
2. Give the ingredients a good stir and then, slowly turn the bowl; running a fork through the avocados. Once you get your desired level of consistency, immediately season it with more of salt, if required. Just before serving; feel free to garnish your recipe with more of fresh cilantro.

NUTRITION

- Calories: 165
- Total Fat: 15g
- Saturated Fat: 2.1g
- Total Carbohydrates: 9.5g

- Dietary Fiber: 6.9g
- Sugars: 1.1g
- Protein: 2.1g

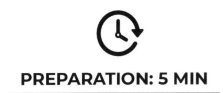

PREPARATION: 5 MIN

COOKING: 30 MIN

SERVES: 4

ROASTED GREEN BEANS

INGREDIENTS

- 3 cups green beans, raw, trimmed
- 1 tablespoon Italian seasoning
- 2 tablespoons olive oil
- Ground black pepper and kosher salt to taste
- 4 tablespoons pumpkin seeds

DIRECTIONS

1. Over moderate heat in a large, frying pan; heat a generous dollop of butter until completely melted.
2. Increase the heat to high and immediately brown the ground beef until almost done, for 5 minutes. Sprinkle with pepper and salt to taste.
3. Decrease the heat to medium; add more of butter and continue to fry the beans in the same pan with the meat for 5 more minutes, stirring frequently.
4. Season the beans with pepper and salt as well. Serve with the leftover butter and add in the optional Crème Fraiche or mayonnaise, if desired.

NUTRITION

- Calories: 155
- Total Fat: 12g
- Saturated Fat: 2.7g
- Total Carbohydrates: 8.7g

- Dietary Fiber: 3.7g
- Sugars: 3.5g
- Protein: 6.4g

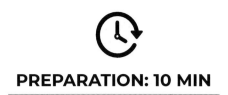

PREPARATION: 10 MIN

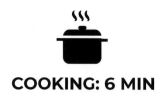

COOKING: 6 MIN

SERVES: 4

FRIED TOFU

INGREDIENTS

- 1 teaspoon seasoning
- 3 tablespoons tamari or soya sauce
- 1 package extra firm tofu (350g)
- ¼ cup nutritional yeast
- 1 tablespoon olive oil

DIRECTIONS

1. Lightly coat a large, non-stick pan with some oil.
2. Put soy sauce (tamari) in a medium sized mixing bowl.
3. Mix the spices together with the yeast in a separate bowl.
4. Slice the tofu into slices, approximately ¼".
5. Dip the tofu pieces in the tamari and then into the yeast mixture.
6. Fry until golden, for 2 to 3 minutes; flip and let the other side to become brown as well, for 2 to 3 more minutes.
7. If required, add a bit of oil.

NUTRITION

- Calories: 139
- Total Fat: 8.6g
- Saturated Fat: 1.4g
- Total Carbohydrates: 5.1g

- Dietary Fiber: 3.1g
- Sugars: 0.9g
- Protein: 12g

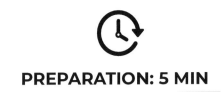

PREPARATION: 5 MIN

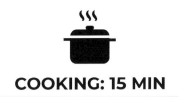

COOKING: 15 MIN

SERVES: 2

CURRY ROASTED CAULIFLOWER

INGREDIENTS

- 1/2 pound cauliflower, approximately a large head; remove the outer leaves, cut into half and then cut out and discard the core; cutting it further into bite-sized pieces
- 2 tablespoons nuts; any of your favorites
- 1 ½ teaspoon curry powder
- 1 tablespoon plus 1 teaspoon extra-virgin olive oil
- 2 teaspoons lemon juice, fresh
- 1 teaspoon kosher salt

DIRECTIONS

1. Preheat your oven to 425°F.
2. Toss the cauliflower pieces with olive oil in a large bowl until evenly coated. Sprinkle with curry powder and salt; give everything a good toss until nicely coated. Spread them out on a large-sized rimmed baking sheet, preferably in an even layer and transfer them to the preheated oven.
3. Roast for 8 to 10 minutes, until the bottom is starting to turn brown. Turn them over and continue to roast for 5 to 7 more minutes, until fork-tender. Place them to the bowl again; toss with the freshly squeezed lemon juice and your favorite nuts. Serve immediately and enjoy.

NUTRITION

- Calories: 188
- Total Fat: 16.7g
- Saturated Fat: 1.8g
- Total Carbohydrates: 8.1g
- Dietary Fiber: 6g
- Sugars: 4.8g
- Protein: 6.3g

PREPARATION: 5 MIN

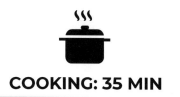

COOKING: 35 MIN

SERVES: 4

ROASTED BRUSSELS SPROUTS WITH PECANS AND ALMOND BUTTER

INGREDIENTS

- 1 pound Brussels sprouts, fresh; ends trimmed
- ¼ cup almond butter
- 2 tablespoons olive oil
- ½ cup pecans, chopped or to taste
- Fresh ground black pepper and salt to taste

DIRECTIONS

1. Using a pastry brush; lightly coat a large-sized roasting pan with 1 tablespoon olive oil and preheat your oven to 350°F in advance.
2. Cut each Brussels sprout lengthwise into halves or fourths.
3. Chop the pecans using a sharp knife and measure the desired amount out.
4. Put the chopped pecans and Brussels sprouts into a large-sized plastic bowl and toss with 1 tablespoon olive oil; generously season with fresh ground black pepper and salt to taste.
5. Arrange the pecans and Brussels sprouts in a single layer on roasting pan. Roast in the preheated oven until the sprouts begin to brown on the edges and are fork-tender, for 30 to 35 minutes, stirring several times during the cooking process.
6. Just before serving, toss the cooked pecans and Brussels sprouts with almond butter. Serve hot and enjoy.

NUTRITION

- Calories: 175
- Total Fat: 23.5g
- Saturated Fat: 3.1g
- Total Carbohydrates: 11g
- Dietary Fiber: 5.7g
- Sugars: 2.9g
- Protein: 7.6g

18. SOUPS

PREPARATION: 10 MIN

COOKING: 30 MIN

SERVES: 4

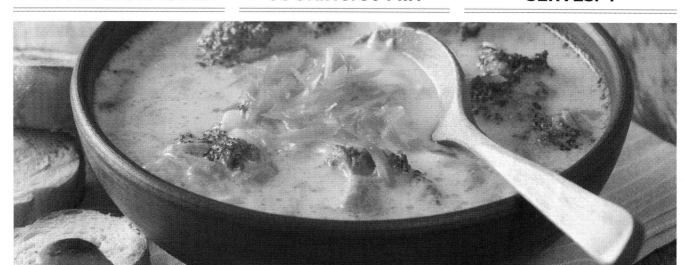

BROCCOLI CHEESE SOUP

INGREDIENTS

- 2 garlic cloves, minced
- ½ cup heavy cream
- 1 ½ cups bone or chicken or vegetable broth
- 2 cups broccoli, cut into florets
- 1 ½ cups cheddar cheese, shredded

DIRECTIONS

1. Over medium heat in a large pot; sauté the garlic until fragrant, for a minute.
2. Add the chicken broth, chopped broccoli and heavy cream. Increase the heat and bring everything together to a boil. Once boiling; decrease the heat and let simmer until the broccoli is tender, for 10 to 20 minutes.
3. Slowly add in the shredded cheddar cheese and continue to cook until melted, stirring constantly, over very low heat settings (if required, work in batches and don't cook over high heat). Once the cheese melts completely; immediately remove the pot from heat. Serve warm and enjoy.

NUTRITION

- Calories: 471
- Total Fat: 38g
- Saturated Fat: 19g
- Total Carbohydrates: 5.7g

- Dietary Fiber: 1.2g
- Sugars: 1.8g
- Protein: 26g

PREPARATION: 5 MIN

COOKING: 55 MIN

SERVES: 4

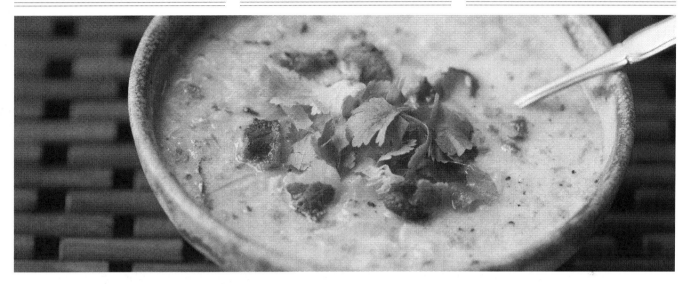

CAULIFLOWER, LEEK, AND BACON SOUP

INGREDIENTS

- 4 cups vegetable or chicken broth
- ½ head of cauliflower; cut into small pieces
- 8 bacon slices
- 1 leek; cut into small pieces
- Pepper and salt to taste

DIRECTIONS

1. Place the leek and cauliflower pieces into a large pot and then fill the pot with chicken broth.
2. Bring it to a boil over moderate heat settings until tender, for 30 to 35 minutes.
3. To create a smooth soup; puree the vegetables using an immersion blender.
4. Microwave the bacon slices on high-heat settings for a minute and then cut into small pieces; dropping the pieces into the soup.
5. Cook for 20 more minutes on low-heat.
6. Add pepper and salt to taste.

NUTRITION

- Calories: 122
- Total Fat: 6.6g
- Saturated Fat: 2g
- Total Carbohydrates: 5.5g
- Dietary Fiber: 2.8g
- Sugars: 2.8g
- Protein: 7.7g

PREPARATION: 5 MIN

COOKING: 15 MIN

SERVES: 2

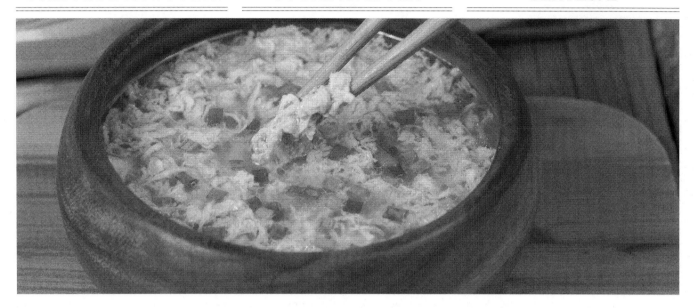

EGG DROP SOUP

INGREDIENTS

- 2 eggs, large
- A pinch of red pepper flakes
- 4 cups bone broth
- 2 tablespoons scallions, sliced
- Freshly ground pepper and salt to taste

DIRECTIONS

1. Scramble the eggs with some fresh pepper in a large bowl; set aside.
2. Now, over high heat settings in a small pot; add bone broth and a pinch of red pepper flakes. Bring it to a boil and then, slowly stir in the egg mixture; continue to mix and bring it to a boil again.
3. Remove from the stove; add pepper and salt to taste
4. Evenly divide the sliced scallions in half; garnish each bowl with it. Enjoy.

NUTRITION

- Calories: 78
- Total Fat: 6.1g
- Saturated Fat: 3.3g
- Total Carbohydrates: 3.5g

- Dietary Fiber: 0.7g
- Sugars: 2.2g
- Protein: 6.1g

PREPARATION: 10 MIN

COOKING: 50 MIN

SERVES: 6

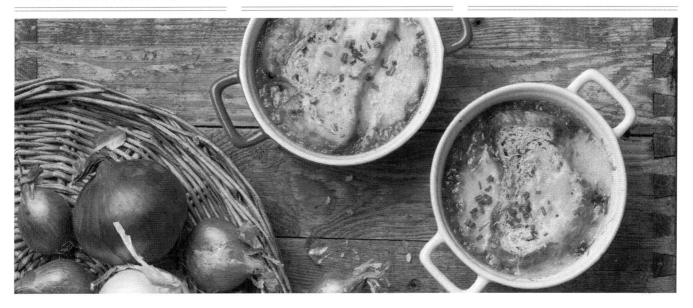

FRENCH ONION SOUP

INGREDIENTS

- 4 drops of erythritol or stevia
- 1 ¼ oz. medium-sized brown onion; chopped
- 5 tablespoons butter
- 3 cups beef stock
- 4 tablespoons olive oil

DIRECTIONS

1. Over medium low heat in a pot; heat the olive oil and butter. Once the butter is melted; add the onions.
2. Cook until the onions turn golden brown, for 20 minutes, uncovered, stirring frequently. Stir in the stevia and cook for 5 more minutes.
3. Add stock to the saucepan; decrease the heat settings to low and let simmer for 25 more minutes.
4. Ladle the soup into separate soup bowls; serve immediately and enjoy.

NUTRITION

- Calories: 219
- Total Fat: 19g
- Saturated Fat: 7.4g
- Total Carbohydrates: 6g
- Dietary Fiber: 1.6g
- Sugars: 4.7g
- Protein: 3.5g

PREPARATION: 10 MIN

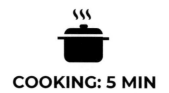
COOKING: 5 MIN

SERVES: 1

CAULIFLOWER FAUX-TATTOOS

INGREDIENTS

- 3 oz. cauliflower; cored and cut into large chunks
- ¼ teaspoon garlic powder
- 1/2 tablespoon butter, optional
- A handful of chives, optional
- 1 cup water
- 1/8 teaspoon each of pepper and salt

DIRECTIONS

1. Add steamer basket/trivet, water and cauliflower to the instant pot.
2. Cover your instant pot with a lid; set the valve to sealing.
3. Select the Manual setting and cook on high pressure for 3 to 5 minutes, less for a firmer mash.
4. Once done; immediately perform a quick release and carefully remove the lid.
5. Carefully remove the inner pot to drain water from and place the cauliflower to an empty and cleaned inner pot.
6. Add butter and the seasonings.
7. Puree the soup using an immersion blender until you get your desired consistency.
8. Give the ingredients a good stir; serve immediately and enjoy.

NUTRITION

- Calories: 87
- Total Fat: 7.6g
- Saturated Fat: 3.9g
- Total Carbohydrates: 3.1g
- Dietary Fiber: 2.1g
- Sugars: 0.8g
- Protein: 1.5g

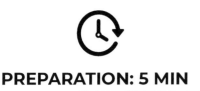

PREPARATION: 5 MIN

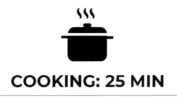

COOKING: 25 MIN

SERVES: 6

THAI SHRIMP SOUP

INGREDIENTS

- 2 tablespoons Butter, unsalted
- ½ pound Medium shrimp, uncooked, peeled and deveined
- ½ White onion, peeled and diced
- 1 tablespoon Minced garlic
- 4 cups Chicken broth
- 2 tablespoons Lime juice
- 2 tablespoons Fish sauce
- 2½ teaspoon Red curry paste
- 1 tablespoon Coconut aminos
- 1 Stalk of lemongrass, chopped
- 1 cup Sliced fresh white mushrooms
- 1 tablespoon Grated ginger
- 1 teaspoon Sea salt
- ½ teaspoon Ground black pepper
- 13.66-ounce Coconut milk, unsweetened, full-fat
- 3 tablespoons Chopped fresh cilantro

DIRECTIONS

1. Switch on the instant pot, add 1 tablespoon butter, press the 'sauté/simmer' button, wait until butter melts, add shrimps, stir well and cook for 3 to 5 minutes or until shrimps turn pink.
2. Transfer shrimps to a plate, add remaining butter and when it melts, add onion and garlic and cook for 3 minutes.
3. Add remaining ingredients, reserving coconut milk, shrimps and cilantro, stir until mixed and press the 'keep warm' button.
4. Shut the instant pot with its lid in the sealed position, then press the 'manual' button, press '+/-' to set the cooking time to 5 minutes and cook at high-pressure setting; when the pressure builds in the pot, the cooking timer will start.
5. When the instant pot buzzes, press the 'keep warm' button, release pressure naturally for 5 minutes, then do a quick pressure release and open the lid.
6. Return shrimps into the instant pot, pour in milk, then press the 'sauté/simmer' button and bring the soup to boil.
7. Press the 'keep warm' button, let soup rest for 2 minutes and then ladle soup into bowls.
8. Garnish the soup with cilantro and serve.

NUTRITION

- Calories: 200
- Fat: 13g
- Protein: 15g
- Net Carbs: 4g
- Fiber: 1g

PREPARATION: 30 MIN

COOKING: 1H 3/4

SERVES: 8

ITALIAN SAUSAGE SOUP WITH TOMATOES & ZUCCHINI NOODLES

INGREDIENTS

- 19.5 oz. pkg Turkey/pork Italian sausage
- 1 tbsp Olive oil
- 8 cups from a carton/can/homemade Chicken stock
- 2 tbsp Tomato paste
- 2 cans/14.5 oz. each Petite tomatoes, diced
- 1 tbsp Dried basil
- 2 tsp Dried Greek oregano
- Optional: 2 tsp Ground fennel
- ½ Green and red bell peppers
- 1/2 medium Onion
- 2x10-inches long Medium zucchini
- Black pepper & salt (as desired)

DIRECTIONS

1. Chop the onions and peppers.
2. Heat a skillet with a bit of oil and add the sausage to cook until it's browned thoroughly.
3. Combine the sausage, tomato paste, diced tomatoes, chicken stock, and spices into the soup pot. Wait for it to simmer.
4. Dice the bell peppers and onion. Sauté them for a few minutes and toss them into the soup. Simmer them using the low-temperature setting (30-60 min.).
5. Prepare the zucchini into noodles using a veggie peeler or spiralizer. Add them to the soup and simmer on low (20-30 min.).
6. Serve them hot, with a portion of freshly grated parmesan as desired

NUTRITION

- Calories: 497
- Net Carbohydrates: 4g
- Protein: 55g

- Fat Content: 27g

PREPARATION: 10 MIN

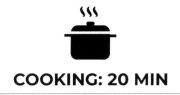

COOKING: 20 MIN

SERVES: 2

SHIRATAKI SOUP

INGREDIENTS

- 2 Boneless, skinless chicken thighs
- 3 cups Chicken stock
- 1 tsp. Minced ginger
- .25 tsp. Cardamom
- 1 Minced garlic clove
- .5 cup Mushrooms
- Optional: 1 tsp. Chili sauce
- 1 pinch Chopped cilantro
- 1 Thinly sliced chili pepper

DIRECTIONS

1. Heat the stock on the stovetop using the med-high temperature setting. Toss in the ginger, garlic, mushrooms, and cardamom. Simmer for about ten minutes.
2. Fold in the chicken and cook until done or about five minutes.
3. Prepare two soup bowls and add the sliced chili pepper to each dish. Serve the soup and garnish with some cilantro.
4. Adjust spices as desired.

NUTRITION

- Calories: 130
- Net Carbohydrates: 1.5g
- Protein: 29.4g

- Fat Content: 12g

PREPARATION: 15 MIN

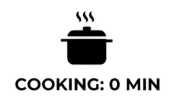

COOKING: 0 MIN

SERVES: 2

CHILLED CUCUMBER SOUP

INGREDIENTS

- 1 cup English cucumber, peeled and chopped
- 1 scallion, chopped
- 2 tablespoons fresh parsley leaves
- 2 tablespoons fresh basil leaves
- ¼ teaspoon fresh lime zest, grated freshly
- 1 cup unsweetened coconut milk
- ¼ cup of water
- ½ tablespoon fresh lime juice
- Salt and ground black pepper, as required

DIRECTIONS

1. Add all the ingredients in a high-speed blender and pulse on high speed until smooth.
2. Transfer the soup into a large serving bowl.
3. Cover the bowl of soup and place in the refrigerator to chill for about 6 hours.
4. Serve chilled.

NUTRITION

- Calories: 198 Cal
- Fat: 10g
- Carbs: 7g

- Protein: 9g
- Fiber: 5g

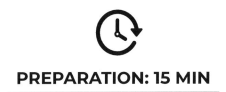

PREPARATION: 15 MIN

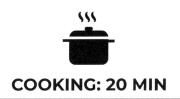

COOKING: 20 MIN

SERVES: 4

CREAMY MUSHROOM SOUP

INGREDIENTS

- 3 tablespoons unsalted butter
- 1 scallion, sliced
- 1 large garlic clove, crushed
- 5 cups fresh button mushrooms, sliced
- 2 cups homemade vegetable broth
- Salt and ground black pepper, as required
- 1 cup heavy cream

DIRECTIONS

1. In a large soup pan, melt the butter over medium heat and sauté the scallion and garlic for about 2-3 minutes.
2. Add the mushrooms cook fry for about 5-6 minutes, stirring frequently.
3. Stir in the broth and bring to a boil.
4. Cook for about 5 minutes.
5. Remove from the heat and with a stick blender, blend the soup until smooth.
6. Return the pan over medium heat.
7. Stir in the cream, salt, and black pepper and cook for about 2-3 minutes, stirring continuously.
8. Remove from the heat and serve hot

NUTRITION

- Calories: 195 Cal
- Fat: 17g
- Carbs: 8g
- Protein: 2g
- Fiber: 5g

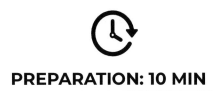
PREPARATION: 10 MIN

COOKING: 15 MIN

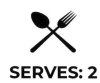
SERVES: 2

BROCCOLI SOUP

INGREDIENTS

- 5 cups homemade chicken broth
- 20 ounces' small broccoli florets
- 12 ounces' cheddar cheese, cubed
- Salt and ground black pepper, as required
- 1 cup heavy cream

DIRECTIONS

1. In a large soup pan, add the broth and broccoli over medium-high heat and bring to a boil.
2. Reduce the heat to low and simmer, covered for about 5-7 minutes.
3. Stir in the cheese and cook for about 2-3 minutes, stirring continuously.
4. Stir in the salt, black pepper, and cream, and cook for about 2 minutes.
5. Serve hot.

NUTRITION

- Calories: 170 Cal
- Fat: 14g
- Carbs: 2g
- Protein: 6g
- Fiber: 3g

19. SALADS

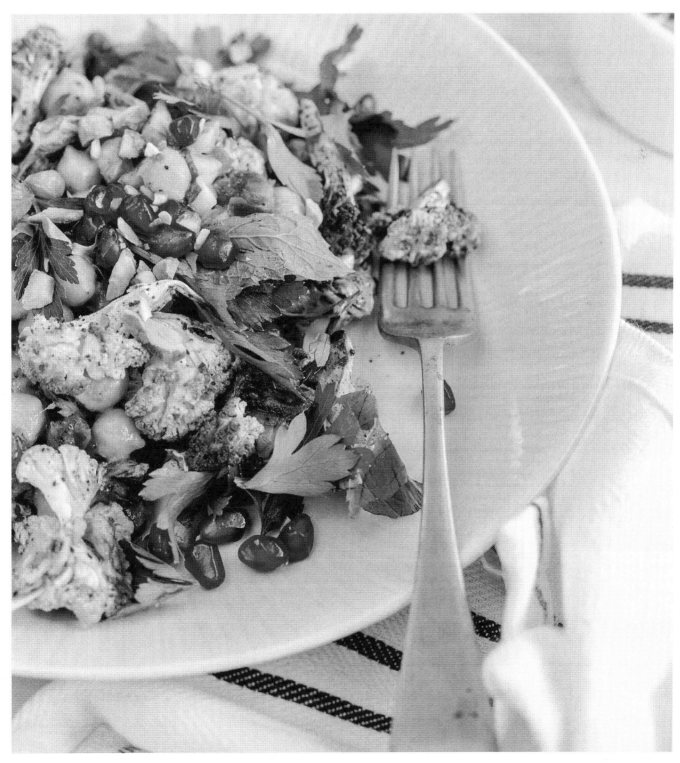

PREPARATION: 10 MIN

COOKING: 10 MIN

SERVES: 2

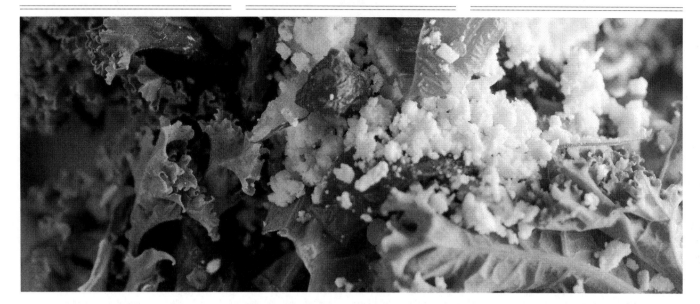

KALE SALAD WITH THE BACON AND BLUE CHEESE

INGREDIENTS

- 4 bacon slices
- 1 tablespoon vinaigrette salad dressing
- 2 cups fresh kale, stemmed and chopped
- Pinch pink Himalayan salt
- Pinch freshly ground black pepper
- ¼ cup pecans
- ¼ cup crumbled blue cheese

DIRECTIONS

1. Add the bacon slices to a skillet over medium-high heat, and fry for 3 t0 4 minutes on each side until evenly crisp.
2. With a slotted spoon, transfer the bacon to a plate lined with paper towels. Set aside to cool.
3. In a large bowl, pour the vinaigrette over the kale and massage it into the kale with your hands. Season with salt and pepper, then allow standing for 5 minutes.
4. Make the salad: Chop the cooked bacon and pecans on your cutting board. Transfer them to the bowl of kale, and top with a sprinkle of blue cheese. Toss the mixture until well blended.
5. To serve, divide the salad between two serving plates.

NUTRITION

- Calories: 328 Cal
- Fat: 19.7g
- Carbs: 5g
- Protein: 8g
- Fiber: 4g

PREPARATION: 10 MIN

COOKING: 0 MIN

SERVES: 2

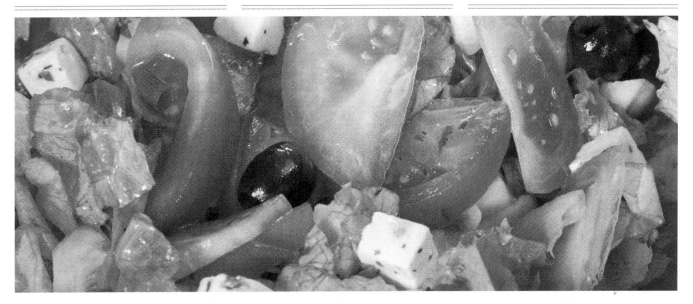

GREEK SALAD WITH VINAIGRETTE SALAD DRESSING

INGREDIENTS

- ½ cup halved grape tomatoes
- 2 cups chopped romaine lettuce
- ¼ cup feta cheese crumbles
- ¼ cup sliced black olives
- 2 tablespoons vinaigrette salad dressing
- Pink Himalayan salt, to taste
- Freshly ground black pepper, to taste
- 1 tablespoon olive oil

DIRECTIONS

1. Make the salad: Stir together the tomatoes, romaine lettuce, feta cheese, olives, and vinaigrette in a large bowl.
2. Sprinkle with salt and pepper, then pour over the olive oil. Toss the salad until well combined.
3. To serve, divide the salad between two serving bowls.

NUTRITION

- Calories: 278 Cal
- Fat: 19.2g
- Carbs: 4.6g
- Protein: 7.3g
- Fiber: 3g

PREPARATION: 20 MIN

COOKING: 0 MIN

SERVES: 4

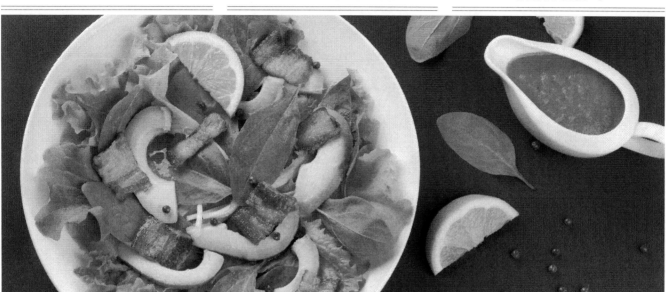

BACON AVOCADO SALAD

INGREDIENTS

- 2 hard-boiled eggs, chopped
- 2 cups spinach
- 2 large avocados, 1 chopped and 1 sliced
- 2 small lettuce heads, chopped
- 1 spring onion, sliced
- 4 cooked bacon slices, crumbled

DIRECTIONS

1. In a large bowl, mix the eggs, spinach, avocados, lettuce, and onion. Set aside.
2. Make the vinaigrette: In a separate bowl, add the olive oil, mustard, and apple cider vinegar. Mix well.
3. Pour the vinaigrette into the large bowl and toss well.
4. Serve topped with bacon slices and sliced avocado.

NUTRITION

- Calories: 268 Cal
- Fat: 16.9g
- Carbs: 8g

- Protein: 5g
- Fiber: 3g

PREPARATION: 10 MIN

COOKING: 5 MIN

SERVES: 4

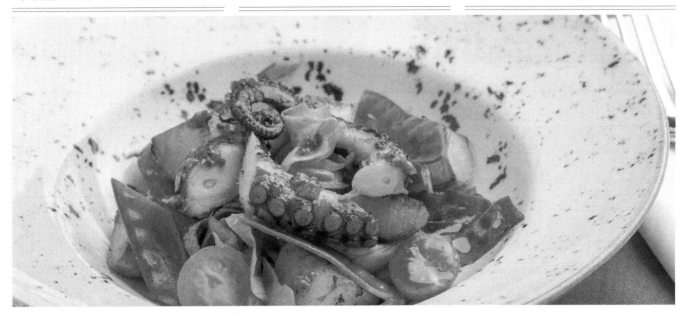

SEARED SQUID SALAD WITH RED CHILI DRESSING

INGREDIENTS

- 4 medium squid tubes, cut into rings
- 1 tablespoon chopped cilantro, for garnish
- Salad:
- 1 cup arugula
- 2 medium cucumbers, halved and cut in strips
- ½ red onion, finely sliced
- ½ cup mint leaves
- ½ cup cilantro leaves, reserve the stems
- Salt and black pepper, to taste
- 2 tablespoons olive oil, divided

DIRECTIONS

1. Make the salad: Mix the arugula, cucumber strips, red onion, mint leaves, and coriander leaves in a salad bowl. Add the salt, pepper, and 1 tablespoon olive oil. Toss to combine well and set aside.
2. Make the dressing: Lightly pound the red chili, garlic clove, and Swerve in a clay mortar with a wooden pestle until it forms a coarse paste. Mix in the lime juice and fish sauce. Set aside.
3. Warm the remaining olive oil in a skillet over high heat. Add the squid and sear for about 5 minutes until lightly browned.
4. Transfer the squid to the salad bowl and top with the dressing. Stir well. Serve garnished with the cilantro.

NUTRITION

- Calories: 278 Cal
- Fat: 24g
- Carbs: 6g
- Protein: 7g
- Fiber: 5g

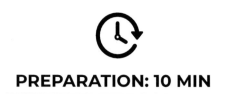

PREPARATION: 10 MIN

COOKING: 5 MIN

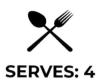

SERVES: 4

CAULIFLOWER AND CASHEW NUT SALAD

INGREDIENTS

- 1 head cauliflower, cut into florets
- ½ cup black olives, pitted and chopped
- 1 cup roasted bell peppers, chopped
- 1 red onion, sliced
- ½ cup cashew nuts
- Chopped celery leaves, for garnish

DIRECTIONS

1. Add the cauliflower into a pot of boiling salted water. Allow to boil for 4 to 5 minutes until fork-tender but still crisp.
2. Remove from the heat and drain on paper towels, then transfer the cauliflower to a bowl.
3. Add the olives, bell pepper, and red onion. Stir well.
4. Make the dressing: In a separate bowl, mix the olive oil, mustard, vinegar, salt, and pepper. Pour the dressing over the veggies and toss to combine.
5. Serve topped with cashew nuts and celery leaves.

NUTRITION

- Calories: 298 Cal
- Fat: 20g
- Carbs: 4g

- Protein: 8g
- Fiber: 3g

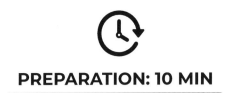
PREPARATION: 10 MIN

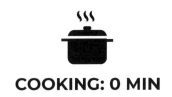
COOKING: 0 MIN

SERVES: 4

SALMON AND LETTUCE SALAD

INGREDIENTS

- 1 tablespoon extra-virgin olive oil
- 2 slices smoked salmon, chopped
- 3 tablespoons mayonnaise
- 1 tablespoon lime juice
- Sea salt, to taste
- 1 cup romaine lettuce, shredded
- 1 teaspoon onion flakes
- ½ avocado, sliced

DIRECTIONS

1. In a bowl, stir together the olive oil, salmon, mayo, lime juice, and salt. Stir well until the salmon is coated fully.
2. Divide evenly the romaine lettuce and onion flakes among four serving plates. Spread the salmon mixture over the lettuce, then serve topped with avocado slices.

NUTRITION

- Calories: 271 Cal
- Fat: 18g
- Carbs: 4g
- Protein: 6g
- Fiber: 3g

PRAWNS SALAD WITH MIXED LETTUCE GREENS

INGREDIENTS

- ½ pound (227g) prawns, peeled and deveined
- Salt and chili pepper, to taste
- 1 tablespoon olive oil
- 2 cups mixed lettuce greens

DIRECTIONS

1. In a bowl, add the prawns, salt, and chili pepper. Toss well.
2. Warm the olive oil over medium heat. Add the seasoned prawns and fry for about 6 to 8 minutes, stirring occasionally, or until the prawns are opaque.
3. Remove from the heat and set the prawns aside on a platter.
4. Make the dressing: In a small bowl, mix the mustard, aioli, and lemon juice until creamy and smooth.
5. Make the salad: In a separate bowl, add the mixed lettuce greens. Pour the dressing over the greens and toss to combine.
6. Divide the salad among four serving plates and serve it alongside the prawns.

NUTRITION

- Calories: 228 Cal
- Fat: 17g
- Carbs: 3g
- Protein: 5g
- Fiber: 8g

PREPARATION: 10 MIN

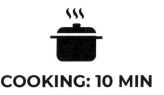

COOKING: 10 MIN

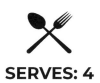

SERVES: 4

POACHED EGG SALAD WITH LETTUCE AND OLIVES

INGREDIENTS

- 4 eggs
- 1 head romaine lettuce, torn into pieces
- ¼ stalk celery, minced
- ¼ cup mayonnaise
- ½ tablespoon mustard
- ½ teaspoon low-carb sriracha sauce
- ¼ teaspoon fresh lime juice
- Salt and black pepper, to taste
- ¼ cup chopped scallions, for garnish
- 10 sliced black olives, for garnish

DIRECTIONS

1. Put the eggs into a pot of salted water over medium heat, then bring to a boil for about 8 minutes.
2. Using a slotted spoon, remove the eggs one at a time from the hot water. Let them cool under running cold water in the sink. When cooled, peel the eggs and slice into bite-sized pieces, then transfer to a large bowl.
3. Make the salad: Add the romaine lettuce, stalk celery, mayo, mustard, sriracha sauce, lime juice, salt, and pepper to the bowl of egg pieces. Toss to combine well.
4. Evenly divide the salad among four serving plates. Serve garnished with scallions and sliced black olives.

NUTRITION

- Calories: 261 Cal
- Fat: 17g
- Carbs: 8g
- Protein: 5.2g
- Fiber: 3.16g

PREPARATION: 10 MIN

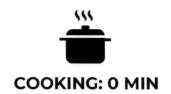
COOKING: 0 MIN

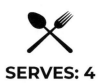
SERVES: 4

REFRESHING CUCUMBER SALAD

INGREDIENTS

- 1/3 cup cucumber basil ranch
- 1 cucumber, chopped
- 3 tomatoes, chopped
- 3 tbsp fresh herbs, chopped
- ½ onion, sliced

DIRECTIONS

1. Add all ingredients into the large mixing bowl and toss well.
2. Serve immediately and enjoy.

NUTRITION

- Calories: 84
- Fat: 3.4g
- Carbs: 12.5g
- Protein: 2g

PREPARATION: 15 MIN

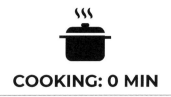

COOKING: 0 MIN

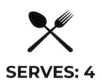

SERVES: 4

CABBAGE COCONUT SALAD

INGREDIENTS

- 1/3 cup unsweetened desiccated coconut
- ½ medium head cabbage, shredded
- 2 tsp sesame seeds
- ¼ cup tamari sauce
- ¼ cup olive oil
- 1 fresh lemon juice
- ½ tsp cumin
- ½ tsp curry powder
- ½ tsp ginger powder

DIRECTIONS

1. Add all ingredients into the large mixing bowl and toss well.
2. Place salad bowl in refrigerator for 1 hour.
3. Serve and enjoy.

NUTRITION

- Calories: 197 Cal
- Fat: 16.6g
- Carbs: 11.4g
- Protein: 3.5g

PREPARATION: 20 MIN

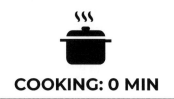

COOKING: 0 MIN

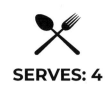

SERVES: 4

AVOCADO CABBAGE SALAD

INGREDIENTS

- 2 avocados, diced
- 4 cups cabbage, shredded
- 3 tbsp fresh parsley, chopped
- 2 tbsp apple cider vinegar
- 4 tbsp olive oil
- 1 cup cherry tomatoes, halved
- 1/2 tsp pepper
- 1 1/2 tsp sea salt

DIRECTIONS

1. Add cabbage, avocados, and tomatoes to a medium bowl and mix well.
2. In a small bowl, whisk together oil, parsley, vinegar, pepper, and salt.
3. Pour dressing over vegetables and mix well.
4. Serve and enjoy.

NUTRITION

- Calories: 253
- Fat: 21.6g
- Carbs: 14g

- Protein: 3.5g

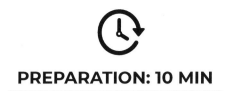
PREPARATION: 10 MIN

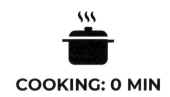
COOKING: 0 MIN

SERVES: 4

TURNIP SALAD

INGREDIENTS

- 4 white turnips, spiralized
- 1 lemon juice
- 4 dill sprigs, chopped
- 2 tbsp olive oil
- 1 1/2 tsp salt

DIRECTIONS

1. Season spiralized turnip with salt and gently massage with hands.
2. Add lemon juice and dill. Season with pepper and salt.
3. Drizzle with olive oil and combine everything well.
4. Serve immediately and enjoy.

NUTRITION

- Calories: 49
- Fat: 1.1g
- Carbohydrates: 9g
- Protein: 1.4g

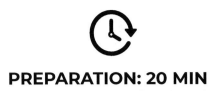

PREPARATION: 20 MIN

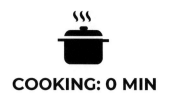

COOKING: 0 MIN

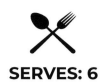

SERVES: 6

BRUSSELS SPROUTS SALAD

INGREDIENTS

- 1 ½ lbs Brussels sprouts, trimmed
- ¼ cup toasted hazelnuts, chopped
- 2 tsp Dijon mustard
- 1 ½ tbsp lemon juice
- 2 tbsp olive oil
- Pepper
- Salt

DIRECTIONS

1. In a small bowl, whisk together oil, mustard, lemon juice, pepper, and salt.
2. In a large bowl, combine together Brussels sprouts and hazelnuts.
3. Pour dressing over salad and toss well.
4. Serve immediately and enjoy.

NUTRITION

- Calories: 111
- Fat: 7.1g
- Carbs: 11g

- Protein: 4.4g

PREPARATION: 10 MIN

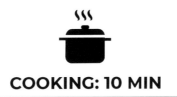

COOKING: 10 MIN

SERVES: 4

BEEF SALAD WITH VEGETABLES

INGREDIENTS

- 1-pound (454g) ground beef
- ¼ cup pork rinds, crushed
- 1 egg, whisked
- 1 onion, grated
- 1 tablespoon fresh parsley, chopped
- ½ teaspoon dried oregano
- 1garlic clove, minced
- Salt and black pepper, to taste
- 2 tablespoons olive oil, divided
- Salad:
- 1 cup chopped arugula
- 1 cucumber, sliced
- 1 cup cherry tomatoes, halved
- 1½ tablespoons lemon juice
- Salt and pepper, to taste

DIRECTIONS

1. Stir together the beef, pork rinds, whisked egg, onion, parsley, oregano, garlic, salt, and pepper in a large bowl until completely mixed.
2. Make the meatballs: On a lightly floured surface, using a cookie scoop to scoop out equal-sized amounts of the beef mixture and form into meatballs with your palm.
3. Heat 1 tablespoon olive oil in a large skillet over medium heat, fry the meatballs for about 4 minutes on each side until cooked through.
4. Remove from the heat and set aside on a plate to cool.
5. In a salad bowl, mix the arugula, cucumber, cherry tomatoes, 1 tablespoon olive oil, and lemon juice. Season with salt and pepper.
6. Make the dressing: In a third bowl, whisk the almond milk, yogurt, and mint until well blended. Pour the mixture over the salad. Serve topped with the meatballs.

NUTRITION

- Calories: 302 Cal
- Fat: 13g
- Carbs: 6g
- Protein: 7g
- Fiber: 4g

PREPARATION: 5 MIN

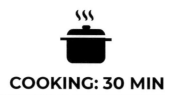
COOKING: 30 MIN

SERVES: 6

NIÇOISE SALAD

INGREDIENTS

- ¾ cup MCT oil
- ½ cup lemon juice
- 1 teaspoon Dijon mustard
- 1 tablespoon fresh thyme leaves, minced
- 1 medium shallot, minced
- 2 teaspoons fresh oregano leaves, minced
- 2 tablespoons fresh basil leaves, minced
- Celtic sea salt and freshly ground black pepper, to taste

DIRECTIONS

1. Melt the butter and heat the olive oil in a nonstick skillet over medium-high heat. Place the tuna steaks in the skillet, and sear for 3 minutes or until opaque, flipping once. Set aside.
2. Make the dressing: Combine all the ingredients for the dressing in a bowl.
3. Make six niçoise salads: Dunk the lettuce and tuna steaks in the dressing bowl to coat well, then arrange the tuna in the middle of the lettuce. Set aside.
4. Blanch the green beans in a pot of boiling salted water for 3 to 5 minutes or until soft but still crisp. Drain and dry with paper towels.
5. Dunk the green beans in the dressing bowl to coat well. Arrange them around the tuna steaks on the lettuce.
6. Top the tuna and green beans with hard-boiled eggs, anchovies, avocado chunks, tomatoes, and olives. Sprinkle 2 tablespoons dressing over each egg, then serve.

NUTRITION

- Calories: 197 Cal
- Fat: 16g
- Carbs: 8g

- Protein: 6g
- Fiber: 4g

SHRIMP, TOMATO, AND AVOCADO SALAD

INGREDIENTS

- 1 pound (454g) shrimp, shelled and deveined
- 2 tomatoes, cubed
- 2 avocados, peeled and cubed
- A handful of fresh cilantro, chopped
- 4green onions, minced
- Juice of 1 lime or lemon
- 1 tablespoon macadamia nut or avocado oil
- Celtic sea salt and fresh ground black pepper, to taste

DIRECTIONS

1. Combine the shrimp, tomatoes, avocados, cilantro, and onions in a large bowl.
2. Squeeze the lemon juice over the vegetables in the large bowl, then drizzle with avocado oil and sprinkle the salt and black pepper to season. Toss to combine well.
3. You can cover the salad, and refrigerate to chill for 45 minutes or serve immediately.

NUTRITION

- Calories: 158 Cal
- Fat: 10g
- Carbs: 4g
- Protein: 9g
- Fiber: 3g

PREPARATION: 4 MIN

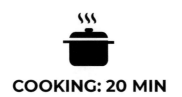
COOKING: 20 MIN

SERVES: 4

PESTO CHICKEN SALAD

INGREDIENTS

- 4 pieces' chicken breast
- .50 cup of pesto
- 1 cup cherry tomatoes
- 3 cups of spinach
- A dash salt
- 3 tbsps. of olive oil

DIRECTIONS

1. For another alternative for plain old, baked chicken, you will want to consider this delicious Pesto chicken salad! To start off, you are going to want to go ahead and prep the stove to 350. As this warms up, place your chicken pieces onto a baking plate and coat with the pepper, salt, and olive oil. When this is done, pop the dish into the oven for forty minutes.
2. When the chicken is cooked through and no longer pink on the inside, you will now take it away from the oven and cool slightly before handling.
3. Once you can handle the chick, you will want to toss it into a bowl along with the pesto and your sliced tomatoes. When the ingredients are mended to your liking, place over a bowl of fresh spinach and enjoy your salad.

NUTRITION

- Calories: 188 Cal
- Fat: 19g
- Carbs: 5g

- Protein: 20g
- Fiber: 3g

PREPARATION: 3 MIN

COOKING: 10 MIN

SERVES: 4

FRESH SUMMER SALAD

INGREDIENTS

- 2 tbsps. of olive oil
- 1 tbsp. of thyme
- 1 tbsp. oregano
- .25 cup of ricotta cheese
- 1 leaf, chopped basil
- 1 tbsp. of balsamic vinegar
- 1 sliced cucumber
- 3 sliced tomatoes
- 5 sliced radishes
- 1 sliced onion

DIRECTIONS

1. Don't be fooled by the name; this salad can be enjoyed at any time of the year! If you are looking for a meatless dish, this is the perfect recipe for you! The first step you will want to take for this recipe will be making your ricotta cheese. You can complete this in a small bowl by mending the thyme, oregano, basil in with the ricotta cheese.
2. Next, you will be making your own dressing! For this task, all you have to do is whisk your vinegar and olive oil together. Once this is complete, season however you would like.
3. Finally, take some time to slice and dice the vegetables according to the directions above. When your veggies are all set, you will want to assemble them in your serving dishes and pour the dressing generously over the top. As a final touch, dollop your ricotta cheese over your salad, and then your salad will be ready for serving.

NUTRITION

- Calories: 158 Cal
- Fat: 19g
- Carbs: 4g
- Protein: 16g
- Fiber: 2g

PREPARATION: 5 MIN

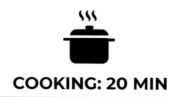

COOKING: 20 MIN

SERVES: 4

KETO TACO SALAD

INGREDIENTS

- 1 lb. ground beef
- 3 tbsp. of olive oil
- A dash pepper
- 1 tbsp. onion powder
- 1 tbsp. cumin
- 1 tbsp. minced garlic clove
- 1 chopped tomato
- .50 cup of sour cream
- .50 cup of black olives
- .25 cup of cheddar cheese
- 2 tbsps. cilantro
- 1 chopped green pepper

DIRECTIONS

1. With taco salad, you will be able to enjoy everything that you love about tacos with a lot fewer carbohydrates! Whether you prepare this for taco Tuesday or a quick lunch, it is sure to be a crowd-pleaser!
2. Start this recipe off by taking out your grilling pan and place it over a moderate temperature. As it warms up, you can add in the olive oil and let that sizzle. When you are set, add in the green pepper, spices, and ground beef. You can also use ground turkey in this recipe if that is more your style. Go ahead and cook these ingredients together for ten minutes or so.
3. When you are all set, place some mixed greens into a bowl and cover with the meat mixture you just created. If you would like some extra flavor, sprinkle some cheddar cheese over the top along with some sour cream.

NUTRITION

- Calories: 138 Cal
- Fat: 27g
- Carbs: 7g
- Protein: 18g
- Fiber: 5g

20. SNACKS

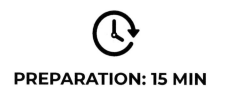
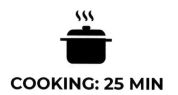

BUNLESS BURGER–KETO STYLE

INGREDIENTS

- 1lb. Ground beef
- 1 tbsp. Worcestershire sauce
- 1 tbsp. Steak Seasoning
- 2 tbsp. Olive oil
- 4 oz. Onions

DIRECTIONS

1. Mix the beef, olive oil, Worcestershire sauce, and seasonings.
2. Grill the burger. Prepare the onions by adding one tablespoon of oil in a skillet to med-low heat. Sauté. Serve.

NUTRITION

- Carbohydrates: 2grams
- Protein: 26grams
- Total Fats: 40grams

- Calories: 479

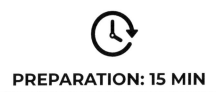

PREPARATION: 15 MIN

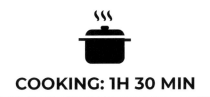

COOKING: 1H 30 MIN

SERVES: 2

SALMON PASTA

INGREDIENTS

- 2 tbsp. Coconut oil
- 2 Zucchinis
- 8 oz. Smoked salmon
- .25 cup Keto-friendly mayo

DIRECTIONS

1. Make noodle-like strands from the zucchini.
2. Warm-up the oil, put the salmon and sauté within 2 to 3 minutes.
3. Stir in the noodles and sauté for 1 to 2 more minutes.
4. Stir in the mayo and serve.

NUTRITION

- Net Carbohydrates: 3grams
- Protein: 21grams
- Total Fats: 42grams
- Calories: 470

PREPARATION: 23 MIN

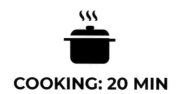

COOKING: 20 MIN

SERVES: 4

WRAPPED BACON CHEESEBURGER

INGREDIENTS

- 7 oz. bacon
- 1 ½ pounds ground beef
- ½ teaspoon salt
- ¼ teaspoon pepper
- 4 oz. cheese, shredded
- 1 head iceberg or romaine lettuce, leaves parted and washed
- 1 tomato, sliced
- ¼ pickled cucumber, finely sliced

DIRECTIONS

1. Cook bacon and set aside.
2. In a separate bowl, combine ground beef, salt, and pepper. Divide mixture into 4 sections, create balls and press each one slightly to form a patty.
3. Put your patties into a frying pan and cook for about 4 minutes on each side.
4. Top each cooked patty with a slice of cheese, several pieces of bacon, and pickled cucumber. Add a bit of tomato.
5. Wrap each burger in a big lettuce leaf.

NUTRITION

- Calories: 684
- Fat: 51grams
- Net Carbs: 5grams

- Protein: 48grams

PREPARATION: 50 MIN

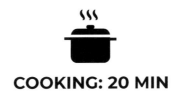

COOKING: 20 MIN

SERVES: 2

KETO TORTILLA CHIPS

INGREDIENTS

- ¼ cube of mozzarella cheese, grated
- ¼ teaspoon cumin powder
- 20grams of almond flour
- 1 teaspoon coriander
- 1 tablespoon cream cheese
- Chili powder, a pinch
- 1 egg
- Salt as per taste

DIRECTIONS

1. Pour the mozzarella cheese, cream cheese, and flour into a microwave-safe bowl and let it melt for 30 seconds. Stir and place again for 30 seconds more.
2. Add spices and egg into the cheese mixture to make the dough.
3. Take two pieces of parchment paper and place dough in a large rectangular form.
4. Remove the parchment paper and place the rectangular dough into a baking dish.
5. Bake it for 15 minutes to 400°F to get one side of the dough brown.
6. Bake the other side of the dough in the same way.
7. Remove the dish from the oven and cut baked dough into rectangular chips.
8. Bake again for 2 minutes to get crunchy chips.

NUTRITION

- Calories: 198
- Fat: 16grams
- Net Carbs: 4grams

- Protein: 11grams

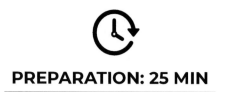

PREPARATION: 25 MIN

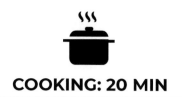

COOKING: 20 MIN

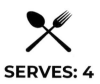

SERVES: 4

CHEESE JALAPENO BREAD

INGREDIENTS

- 4 eggs
- 1/3 cup coconut flour
- ¼ cup of water
- ¼ cup butter
- ¼ teaspoon pepper
- 3 jalapeno chilies, chopped
- ¼ teaspoon onion powder
- ½ cup cheddar cheese, grated
- ¼ cup parmesan cheese, grated
- ¼ teaspoon baking powder, gluten-free
- ½ teaspoon garlic powder
- ½ teaspoon salt

DIRECTIONS

1. Preheat the oven to 400° F.
2. In a bowl, mix together eggs, pepper, salt, water, and butter.
3. Add baking powder, garlic powder, onion powder, and coconut flour and mix well.
4. Add jalapenos, cheddar cheese, and parmesan cheese. Mix well and season with pepper.
5. Line baking tray with parchment pepper.
6. Pour batter into a baking tray and spread evenly.
7. Bake for 15 minutes.
8. Slice and serve.

NUTRITION

- Calories: 249
- Fat: 22grams
- Net Carbs: 2.7grams

- Protein: 11.1grams

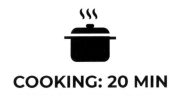

KETO SEED CRACKERS

INGREDIENTS

- 2 ½ cups water
- 10grams of pumpkin seeds
- ½ tablespoon of Psyllium husk powder
- 10grams flax seeds
- Salt as per taste 10grams sesame seeds
- ¼ cup sunflower seeds

DIRECTIONS

1. Preheat oven to 360° F and grease the baking dish.
2. Pour water in a bowl and add whisk powder. Stir well powder in the water to remove all lumps.
3. Later on, add salt and all seeds into the water. You can increase or decrease the quantity of water according to your seeds and set aside for a few minutes to get a gel shape mixture.
4. Make a thin layer of gel mixture in the baking dish and let it bake for 30 minutes.
5. After the fixed time, cut the gel mixture with a sharp knife to make the shape of crackers.
6. Put them back and let it bake for 45 minutes. After the timer alarms you, check out the crisp of the crackers.
7. Serve it as a snack along with your meal.

Tips:
- Do not pour powder first and then water in the bowl. You need to pour the powder in the water instead of water in the powder.
- You can place a silicone mat in the baking dish to avoid the sticking of the mixture.
- You can change the number of seeds as per your choice.
- Carefully use husk powder due to its gel nature. You should make the gel mixture thin to get the best results.

NUTRITION

- Calories: 130
- Fat: 10grams
- Net Carbs: 6grams

- Protein: 3grams

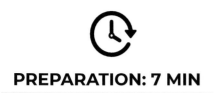

PREPARATION: 7 MIN

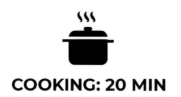

COOKING: 20 MIN

SERVES: 2

KETO COCONUT PORRIDGE

INGREDIENTS

- 4 tablespoons coconut flour
- 2 eggs, beaten
- 4 tablespoons golden flax meal
- 2 tablespoons butter
- ½ cup of water 2 tablespoons coconut cream
- Salt as per taste 2 tablespoon sweetener, any low carb

DIRECTIONS

1. Pour water, salt, flax meal and coconut flour in a pot and stir on medium heat. Continue whisking to make it thicken.
2. Lower the flame; add beaten egg slowly while stirring. Remove from the heat.
3. Add butter, sweetener, and cream in the porridge and whisk.
4. The coconut flour porridge is ready for your morning meal. Top it with your favorite topping items like berries, chocolate chips, or hazelnuts.

NUTRITION

- Calories: 345
- Fat: 28.5grams
- Net Carbs: 13grams
- Protein: 13grams

PREPARATION: 25 MIN

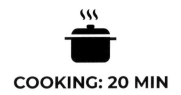

COOKING: 20 MIN

SERVES: 2

DAIRY-FREE PIZZA

INGREDIENTS

- 4 eggs
- 2 cups cauliflower, grated
- 2 tablespoons coconut flour
- 1 tablespoon Psyllium husk powder
- 2 pinches salt
- Smoked salmon
- Avocado
- Spinach
- Herbs

DIRECTIONS

1. Heat the oven to 350° F and line the pizza tray with parchment.
2. Take a mixing bowl and place the eggs, cauliflower, coconut flour, and Psyllium husk powder into it. Mix all the ingredients, add salt, and leave for 5 minutes until the mixture thickens up.
3. Pour your base for the breakfast pizza onto the tray.
4. Bake your pizza for 15 minutes.
5. Remove it and decorate with smoked salmon, avocado, spinach, and herbs.

NUTRITION

- Calories: 226
- Fat: 55grams
- Net Carbs: 7grams

- Protein: 15grams

PREPARATION: 15 MIN

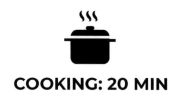

COOKING: 20 MIN

SERVES: 2

LOW CARB BANANA WAFFLES

INGREDIENTS

- ½ banana, mashed
- Coconut oil, for frying
- 1 egg, beaten
- 3 to 4 drops of vanilla extract
- 25g almond flour
- ¼ teaspoon baking powder
- 50ml coconut milk
- Salt to taste
- 1 teaspoon Psyllium husk powder
- Grounded cinnamon, a pinch

DIRECTIONS

1. Take a bowl and beat the egg well.
2. Add mashed banana, flour, coconut milk, husk powder, cinnamon, salt, vanilla extract, and baking powder and mix well. Set aside the mixture.
3. Heat the oil and pour the mixture in the pan.
4. Fry and dish out the waffles.
5. Serve it with coconut cream and chocolate chips.

Tip: Take a can of coconut milk and set for 4 hours in a refrigerator to separate the water and cream. Scoop out the cream from the can and beat the cream for a few minutes. Whipped coconut cream is ready to serve with waffles.

NUTRITION

- Calories: 155
- Fat: 13grams
- Net Carbs: 4grams

- Protein: 5grams

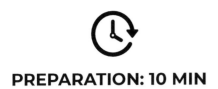

PREPARATION: 10 MIN

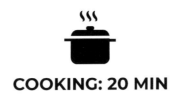

COOKING: 20 MIN

SERVES: 4

AVOCADO YOGURT DIP

INGREDIENTS

- 2 avocados
- 1 lime juice
- 3 garlic cloves, minced
- ½ cup Greek yogurt
- Pepper
- Salt

DIRECTIONS

1. Scoop out avocado flesh using the spoon and place it in a bowl.
2. Mash avocado flesh using the fork.
3. Add remaining ingredients and stir to combine.
4. Serve and enjoy.

NUTRITION

- Calories: 139
- Fat: 11grams
- Net Carbs: 9grams

- Protein: 4grams

PREPARATION: 10 MIN

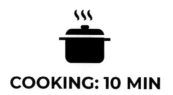
COOKING: 10 MIN

SERVES: 4

CHEESE BALLS

INGREDIENTS

- ½ cup pistachios, de-shelled
- 4 oz. goat cheese
- 4 sun-dried tomatoes
- Salt to taste

DIRECTIONS

1. Lightly crush the pistachios using a mortar and pestle (don't grind).
2. Sprinkle the crushed pistachios with salt to taste.
3. Chop dried tomatoes and cut goat cheese into 4 slices.
4. Form goat cheese into balls with dried tomatoes.
5. Cover the sun-dried tomato goat cheese balls by rolling them around the pistachio mixture.
6. Once covered, roll the balls again into the leftover dust of pistachio.
7. Serve immediately and enjoy.

NUTRITION

- Calories: 162
- Total Fat: 13g
- Saturated Fat: 5g
- Total Carbohydrates: 4.2g
- Dietary Fiber: 1.6g
- Sugars: 1.2g
- Protein: 8.5g

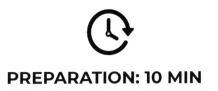

PREPARATION: 10 MIN

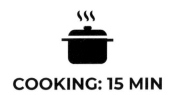

COOKING: 15 MIN

SERVES: 4

SPICY CHICKEN THIGHS

INGREDIENTS

- 1 pound chicken thighs, boneless
- A small handful of fresh cilantro, for garnish
- ½ tablespoon chili powder
- Lime wedges, fresh for serving
- ½ tablespoon extra-virgin olive oil, organic
- Fresh ground pepper and sea salt to taste

DIRECTIONS

1. Preheat your oven to 375°F.
2. Place the chicken thighs on a sheet pan, and drizzle with the olive oil; turn several times until evenly coated with the oil. Now, rub the chicken pieces with chili powder, pepper, and salt.
3. Roast the chicken thighs for 12 to 15 minutes, until cooked through.
4. Sprinkle with fresh cilantro; serve immediately with some lime wedges and enjoy.

NUTRITION

- Calories: 246
- Total Fat: 13g
- Saturated Fat: 3.8g
- Total Carbohydrates: 2.3g
- Dietary Fiber: 0.8g
- Sugars: 0.4g
- Protein: 19g

PREPARATION: 5 MIN

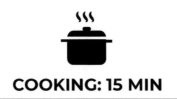
COOKING: 15 MIN

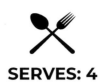
SERVES: 4

CORNED BEEF AND CAULIFLOWER HASH

INGREDIENTS

- 2 cups chopped raw cauliflower
- ½ cup onion, chopped
- 2 cups chopped corned beef
- 1 tablespoon extra-virgin olive oil
- Pepper and salt to taste

DIRECTIONS

1. Over moderate heat in a medium-sized sauté pan; heat the olive oil until hot. Carefully, add the corned beef and cook until the fat renders out, for a couple of minutes.
2. Add the raw cauliflower and continue to cook until caramelized, for 6 to 8 minutes, stirring every now and then. Add and cook the onions until slightly browned and softened, for more 5 minutes.
3. Season with pepper and salt to taste. Serve immediately and enjoy.

NUTRITION

- Calories: 275
- Total Fat: 19g
- Saturated Fat: 5.9g
- Total Carbohydrates: 4.4g
- Dietary Fiber: 1.4g
- Sugars: 1.8
- Protein: 18g

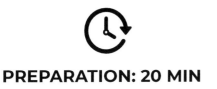

PREPARATION: 20 MIN

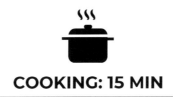

COOKING: 15 MIN

SERVES: 2

LOW CARB GNOCCHI

INGREDIENTS

- 3 egg yolks, large
- ½ teaspoon garlic powder
- 2 cups mozzarella, low moisture, shredded, park skim
- 1 teaspoon salt

DIRECTIONS

1. Sprinkle mozzarella with the seasonings and then melt it in a toaster oven for 10 minutes, stirring every now and then. Separate the egg yolks from whites and beat them until combined well.
2. Combine the melted mozzarella with half of the egg yolks mixture using two silicone spatulas.
3. Once everything is combined well, separate it into ¼; rolling each fourth into a thin and long strip on a parchment paper piece.
4. Cut approximately 1" pieces in every strip until you have plenty of cheese gnocchi. To make them look like more traditional gnocchi; gently press a fork onto them.
5. Fill a pot with water and bring it to a boil, over moderate heat; carefully drop the pieces of gnocchi into the boiling water. Boil them until starts floating and then drain.
6. The next step is to fry the gnocchi on an oiled pan on both sides. Enjoy.

NUTRITION

- Calories: 440
- Total Fat: 32g
- Saturated Fat: 19g
- Total Carbohydrates: 3.9g

- Dietary Fiber: 0.1g
- Sugars: 2.2g
- Protein: 29g

PREPARATION: 10 MIN

COOKING: 8 MIN

SERVES: 3

AVOCADO FRIES

INGREDIENTS

- For Fries:
- 1 ½ cups almond meal
- 1 large egg
- 3 ripe avocados
- 1 ½ cups sunflower oil
- Cayenne pepper and salt to taste
- For Spicy Mayo, Optional:
- 1 teaspoon Sriracha
- 2 tablespoons homemade mayonnaise

DIRECTIONS

1. Break and beat the egg in a large sized mixing bowl. Combine the almond meal with a small amount of cayenne pepper and salt in a separate bowl.
2. Over moderate heat in a deep pan; heat plenty oil until bubbles arise. Coat each of the avocado slices into the beaten egg and then roll the coated slice into the prepared almond meal; ensure that the slices are evenly coated with the mixture.
3. To avoid splashing; carefully lower every slice of avocado into the hot pan.
4. Fry each piece until turn light brown, for 30 to 50 seconds. To soak up the excess oil; line a large plate with paper towels and quickly transfer the fried slices to the large plate. Serve hot with the optional sauce and enjoy.
5. For the Optional Spicy Mayo: Combine some mayo with the Sriracha sauce in a medium-sized bowl; mix well.

NUTRITION

- Calories: 670
- Total Fat: 59g
- Saturated Fat: 6.9g
- Total Carbohydrates: 8g

- Dietary Fiber: 12g
- Sugars: 3.8g
- Protein: 18g

21. DESSERTS

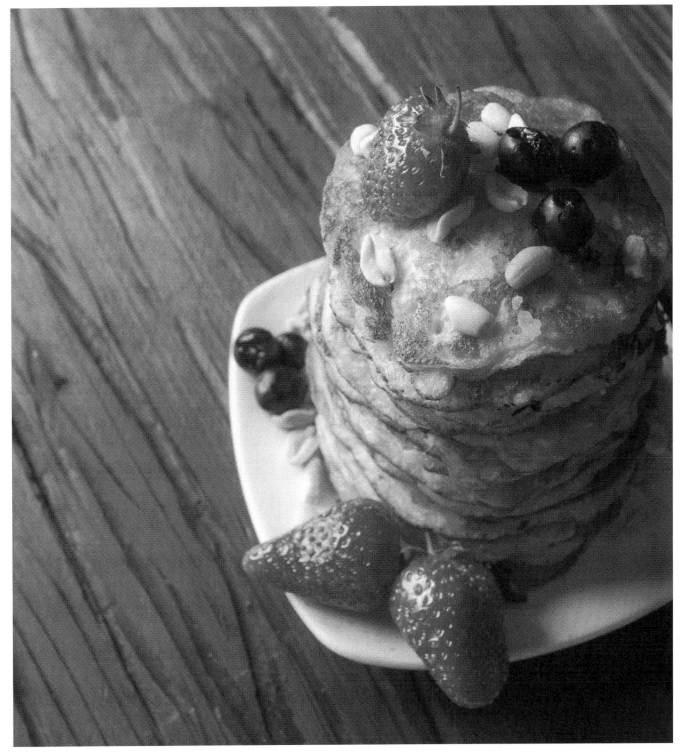

PREPARATION: 2H 35 MIN

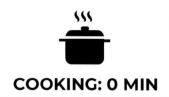

COOKING: 0 MIN

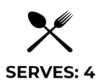

SERVES: 4

MOCHA MOUSSE

INGREDIENTS

- For the Cream Cheese:
- 8 ounces Cream cheese, softened and full-fat
- 3 tablespoons Sour cream, full-fat
- 2 tablespoons Butter, softened
- 1 ½ teaspoons Vanilla extract, unsweetened
- 1/3 cup Erythritol
- ¼ cup Cocoa powder, unsweetened
- 3 teaspoons Instant coffee powder
- For the Whipped Cream:
- 2/3 cup Heavy whipping cream, full-fat
- 1 ½ teaspoon Erythritol
- ½ teaspoon Vanilla extract, unsweetened

DIRECTIONS

1. Prepare cream cheese mixture: For this, place cream cheese in a bowl, add sour cream and butter then beat until smooth.
2. Now add erythritol, cocoa powder, coffee, and vanilla and blend until incorporated, set aside until required.
3. Prepare whipping cream: For this, place whipping cream in a bowl and beat until soft peaks form.
4. Beat in vanilla and erythritol until stiff peaks form, then add 1/3 of the mixture into cream cheese mixture and fold until just mixed.
5. Then add remaining whipping cream mixture and fold until evenly incorporated.
6. Spoon the mousse into a freezer-proof bowl and place in the refrigerator for 2 ½ hours until set.
7. Serve straight away.

NUTRITION

- Calories: 421.7
- Fat: 42g
- Protein: 6g

- Net Carbs: 6.5g
- Fiber: 2g

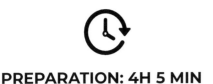

PREPARATION: 4H 5 MIN

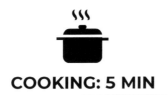

COOKING: 5 MIN

SERVES: 5

STRAWBERRY RHUBARB CUSTARD

INGREDIENTS

- 27 ounces Coconut milk, full-fat
- 2 Eggs
- ¾ cup Strawberries, fresh
- ½ cup Rhubarb, chopped
- ¼ cup Collagen, grass-fed
- 1 teaspoon Vanilla extract, unsweetened
- 1/16 teaspoon Stevia, liquid
- 1/16 teaspoon Salt
- 1 ½ tablespoons Gelatin, grass-fed
- 1 cup Water

DIRECTIONS

1. Place all the ingredients in a food processor except for the gelatin and water, pulse until smooth, then add gelatin and blend until smooth.
2. Divide the custard evenly between five half-pint jars and cover with their lid.
3. Switch on the instant pot, pour in water, insert trivet stand, place jars on it and shut the instant pot with its lid the in the sealed position.
4. Press the 'manual' button, press '+/-' to set the cooking time to 5 minutes and cook at high-pressure setting; when the pressure builds in the pot, the cooking timer will start.
5. When the instant pot buzzes, press the 'keep warm' button, do a quick pressure release and open the lid.
6. Carefully remove the jars, let them cool at room temperature for 15 minutes or more until they can be comfortably picked up.
7. Then transfer the custard jars into the refrigerator for a minimum of 4 hours and cool completely.
8. When ready to serve, shake the jars a few times to mix all the ingredients and then serve.

NUTRITION

- Calories: 262
- Fat: 24g
- Protein: 5g
- Net Carbs: 3g
- Fiber: 3g

PREPARATION: 4H 25 MIN

COOKING: 9 MIN

SERVES: 6

CRÈME BRULEE

INGREDIENTS

- 2 cups Heavy whipping cream
- 6 Egg yolks
- 5 tablespoons Erythritol sweetener
- 1 tablespoon Vanilla extract, unsweetened
- 1 cup Water

DIRECTIONS

1. Place all the ingredients in a large bowl, reserving 2 tablespoons sweetener and water, and whisk well until combined.
2. Evenly divide the mixture among six ramekins and then cover each ramekin with aluminum foil.
3. Switch on the instant pot, pour in water, then insert trivet stand and stack ramekins on it.
4. Shut the instant pot with its lid in the sealed position, then press the 'manual' button, press '+/-' to the set the cooking time to 9 minutes and cook at high-pressure setting; when the pressure builds in the pot, the cooking timer will start.
5. When the instant pot buzzes, press the 'keep warm' button, release pressure naturally for 15 minutes, then do a quick pressure release and open the lid.
6. Take out the ramekins, uncover them, let rest for 15 minutes at room temperature and then cool completely in the refrigerator for 4 hours.
7. When ready to serve, sprinkle 1 teaspoon of remaining sweetener over each crème Brulee and burn the sweetener by using a hand torch.
8. Serve straight away.

NUTRITION

- Calories: 500
- Fat: 51g
- Protein: 6g

- Net Carbs: 5g
- Fiber: 0g

PREPARATION: 4H 25 MIN

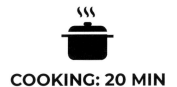

COOKING: 20 MIN

SERVES: 4

PUMPKIN PIE PUDDING

INGREDIENTS

- 2 Eggs
- 1 cup Heavy whipping cream, divided
- 3/4 cup Erythritol sweetener
- 15 ounces Pumpkin puree
- 1 teaspoon Pumpkin pie spice
- 1 teaspoon Vanilla extract, unsweetened
- 1 ½ cup Water

DIRECTIONS

1. Crack eggs in a bowl, add ½ cup cream, sweetener, pumpkin puree, pumpkin pie spice, and vanilla and whisk until blended.
2. Take a 6 by 3-inch baking pan, grease it well with avocado oil, then pour in egg mixture, smooth the top and cover with aluminum foil.
3. Switch on the instant pot, pour in water, insert a trivet stand and place baking pan on it.
4. Shut the instant pot with its lid in the sealed position, then press the 'manual' button, press '+/-' to the set the cooking time to 20 minutes and cook at high-pressure setting; when the pressure builds in the pot, the cooking timer will start.
5. When the instant pot buzzes, press the 'keep warm' button, release pressure naturally for 10 minutes, then do a quick pressure release and open the lid.
6. Take out the baking pan, uncover it, let cool for 15 minutes at room temperature, then transfer the pan into the refrigerator for 4 hours or until cooled.
7. Top pie with remaining cream, then cut it into slices and serve.

NUTRITION

- Calories: 184
- Fat: 16g
- Protein: 3g
- Net Carbs: 5g
- Fiber: 2g

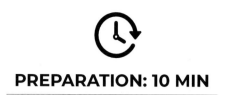

PREPARATION: 10 MIN

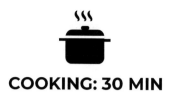

COOKING: 30 MIN

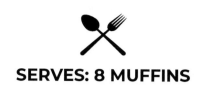

SERVES: 8 MUFFINS

CHOCOLATE MUFFINS

INGREDIENTS

- 2 cups Pumpkin, chopped, steamed
- 1/2 cup Coconut flour
- 1/8 teaspoon Salt
- 4 tablespoons Erythritol sweetener
- 1 cup Cacao powder, unsweetened
- 1/2 cup Collagen protein powder
- 1 teaspoon Baking soda
- 4.6 ounces Cacao butter, melted
- 1/2 cup Avocado oil
- 2 teaspoons Apple cider vinegar
- 3 teaspoons Vanilla extract, unsweetened
- 3 Eggs, pastured

DIRECTIONS

1. Set oven to 350 degrees F and let preheat until muffins are ready to bake.
2. Add all the ingredients in a food processor or blender, except for collagen, and pulse for 1 to 2 minutes or until well combined and incorporated.
3. Then add collagen and pulse at low speed until just mixed.
4. Take an eight cups silicon muffin tray, grease the cups with avocado oil and then evenly scoop the prepared batter in them.
5. Place the muffin tray into the oven and bake the muffins for 30 minutes or until thoroughly cooked and a knife inserted into each muffin comes out clean.
6. When done, let muffins cool in the pan for 10 minutes, then take them out from the tray and cool on the wire rack.
7. Place muffins in a large freezer bag or wrap each muffin with a foil and store them in the refrigerator for four days or in the freezer for up to 3 months.
8. When ready to serve, microwave muffins for 45 seconds to 1 minute or until thoroughly heated and then serve with coconut cream.

NUTRITION

- Calories: 111
- Fat: 9.9g
- Protein: 2.8g

- Net Carbs: 3g
- Fiber: 1g

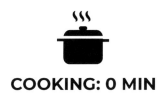
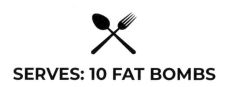
LEMON FAT BOMBS

INGREDIENTS

- 3/4 cup Coconut butter, full-fat
- 1/4 cup Avocado oil
- 3 tablespoons Lemon juice
- Zest of 1 lemon
- 1 tablespoon Coconut cream, full-fat
- 1 tablespoon Erythritol sweetener
- 1 teaspoon Vanilla extract, unsweetened
- 1/8 teaspoon Salt

DIRECTIONS

1. Place all the ingredients for fat bombs in a blender and pulse until well combined.
2. Take a baking dish, line it with parchment sheet, then transfer the fat bomb mixture on the sheet and place the sheet into the freezer for 45 minutes until firm enough to shape into balls.
3. Then remove the baking sheet from the freezer, roll the fat bomb mixture into ten balls, and arrange the fat bombs on the baking sheet in a single layer.
4. Return the baking sheet into the freezer, let chilled until hard and set, and then store in the freezer for up to 2 months.
5. Serve when required.

NUTRITION

- Calories: 164
- Fat: 16.7g
- Protein: 1.3g
- Net Carbs: 0.4g
- Fiber: 3g

PREPARATION: 6H 10 MIN

COOKING: 0 MIN

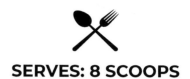

SERVES: 8 SCOOPS

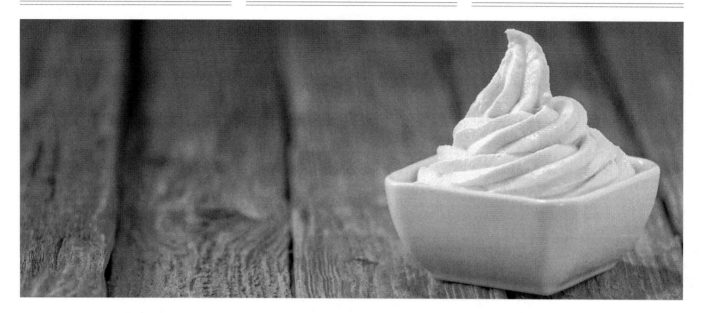

VANILLA FROZEN YOGURT

INGREDIENTS

- 1 cup Yogurt, organic, full-fat, chilled
- 4 tablespoons Erythritol sweetener
- 1 tablespoon MCT oil
- 2 teaspoons Vanilla extract, unsweetened
- 1 tablespoon Lime juice

DIRECTIONS

1. Add all the ingredients in a blender or food processor and pulse for 1 to 2 minutes or until smooth and creamy
2. Then pour the yogurt mixture into a large meal prep glass container and store in the freezer for 5 to 6 hours until hard and for up to 3 to 4 months.
3. When ready to serve, let yogurt rest at room temperature for 15 to 20 minutes or until slightly soft and then scoop into bowls.

NUTRITION

- Calories: 122
- Fat: 11.4g
- Protein: 3.2g
- Net Carbs: 2.7g
- Fiber: 0g

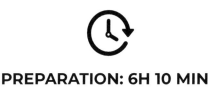

PREPARATION: 6H 10 MIN

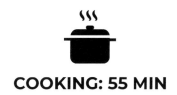

COOKING: 55 MIN

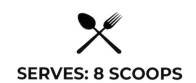

SERVES: 8 SCOOPS

ICE CREAM

INGREDIENTS

- 1/3 cup Erythritol sweetener
- 3 tablespoons Butter, grass-fed, unsalted
- 1/4 cup MCT oil
- 1 teaspoon Vanilla extract, unsweetened
- 3 cups Heavy cream, full-fat

DIRECTIONS

1. Place a large saucepan over medium, add butter and cook for 3 to 5 minutes or until butter melts.
2. Add 2 cups cream and sweetener, stir well, bring the mixture to boil, then reduce heat to medium-low level and simmer the mixture for 30 to 45 minutes or until reduced by half and thickened enough to coat the back of a spoon.
3. Then pour the ice cream mixture into a large bowl and let it cool at the room temperature.
4. Add MCT oil and vanilla, stir until mixed and whisk in remaining cream until smooth.
5. Pour the mixture into a large meal prep container, smooth the top with a spatula and let it freeze for 5 to 6 hours or until firm, stirring the ice cream every 30 minutes in the first two hours and every 1 hour for the next 2 to 3 hours.
6. Then shut the container with its lid and store the ice cream for 3 to 4 months.
7. When ready to serve, let ice cream rest at room temperature for 15 to 20 minutes or until soften and then scoop into bowls.

NUTRITION

- Calories: 347
- Fat: 36g
- Protein: 2g

- Net Carbs: 3g
- Fiber: 0g

PREPARATION: 10 MIN

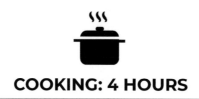

COOKING: 4 HOURS

SERVES: 8

RASPBERRY MOUSSE

INGREDIENTS

- 3 oz. fresh raspberry
- 2 cups heavy whipping cream
- 2 oz. pecans, chopped
- ¼ tsp. vanilla extract
- ½ lemon, the zest

DIRECTIONS

1. Pour the whipping cream into the dish and blend until it becomes soft.
2. Put the lemon zest and vanilla into the dish and mix thoroughly.
3. Put the raspberries and nuts into the cream mix and stir well.
4. Cover the dish with plastic wrap and put it in the fridge for 3 hours.
5. Top with raspberries and serve.

NUTRITION

- Carbohydrates: 3g
- Fat: 26g
- Protein: 2g

- Calories: 255

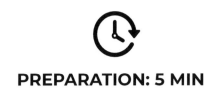

PREPARATION: 5 MIN

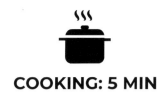

COOKING: 5 MIN

SERVES: 6

CHOCOLATE SPREAD WITH HAZELNUTS

INGREDIENTS

- 2 Tbsp. cacao powder
- 5 oz. hazelnuts, roasted and without shells
- 1 oz. unsalted butter
- ¼ cup coconut oil

DIRECTIONS

1. Whisk all the spread ingredients with a blender for as long as you want. Remember, the longer you blend, the smoother your spread.

NUTRITION

- Carbohydrates: 2g
- Fat: 28g
- Protein: 4g

- Calories: 271

PREPARATION: 20 MIN

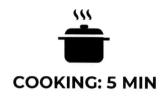

COOKING: 5 MIN

SERVES: 2

QUICK AND SIMPLE BROWNIE

INGREDIENTS

- 3 Tbsp. Keto chocolate chips
- 1 Tbsp. unsweetened cacao powder
- 2 Tbsp. salted butter
- 2¼ Tbsp. powdered sugar

DIRECTIONS

1. Combine 2 Tbsp. of chocolate chips and butter, melt them in a microwave for 10-15 minutes. Add the remaining chocolate chips, stir and make a sauce.
2. Add the cacao powder and powdered sugar to the sauce and whisk well until you have a dough.
3. Place the dough on a baking sheet, form the Brownie.
4. Put your Brownie into the oven (preheated to 350°F).
5. Bake for 5 minutes.

NUTRITION

- Carbohydrates: 9g
- Fat: 30g
- Protein: 13g

- Calories: 100

PREPARATION: 20 MIN

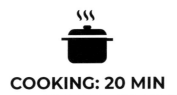

COOKING: 20 MIN

SERVES: 18

CUTE PEANUT BALLS

INGREDIENTS

- 1 cup salted peanuts, chopped
- 1 cup peanut butter
- 1 cup powdered sweetener
- 8 oz. keto chocolate chips

DIRECTIONS

1. Combine the chopped peanuts, peanut butter, and sweetener in a separate dish. Stir well and make a dough. Divide it into 18 pieces and form small balls. Put them in the fridge for 10-15 minutes.
2. Use a microwave to melt your chocolate chips.
3. Plunge each ball into the melted chocolate.
4. Return your balls in the fridge. Cool for about 20 minutes.

NUTRITION

- Carbohydrates: 7g
- Fat: 17g
- Protein: 7g

- Calories: 194

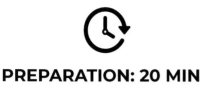
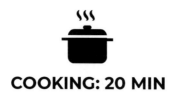

TURKEY CARROT MUSHROOM DUMPLINGS

INGREDIENTS

- 3/4 carrots finely julienned
- 1 pound ground turkey
- 1/2 c. mushrooms finely chopped
- 2 tablespoons soy sauce
- 1 tablespoon rice wine
- 1 tablespoon sesame oil
- 1/2 tablespoon onion powder
- 1/8 of a tablespoon salt
- 2 tablespoons cornstarch
- 30 dumpling wrappers

DIRECTIONS

1. In a microwaveable dish, place the carrots and cover them with water. Cook until soft, depending on how finely chopped the carrots are, for around 3 minutes. Let it drain and cool.
2. Mix the cooked vegetables, turkey, mushrooms, soy sauce, rice vinegar, sesame seed, onion powder, salt, and cornstarch together in a wide dish. Together, stir when well mixed.
3. Spoon onto a dumpling wrapper, a well-shaped teaspoon of filling. Seal with wrapper filling. Cover the extra dumplings.
4. Bring water to the bottom of the steamer pot to boil. Place the dumplings in a steamer lined with parchment paper. Steam for 15 minutes, until cooked.

NUTRITION

- Calories: 48
- Fat (0g sat): 1g
- Protein: 3g
- Carb: 4g
- Sodium: 87mg

PREPARATION: 5 MIN

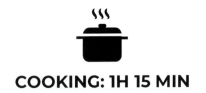

COOKING: 1H 15 MIN

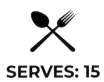

SERVES: 15

LEMON BREAD FROM STARBUCKS

INGREDIENTS

- 6 eggs
- 2 tbsp. unchilled cream cheese
- 9 tbsp. butter
- 1 tsp. vanilla
- 2 tbsp. heavy whipping cream
- ½ tsp. of salt
- 2/3 cup Monkfruit Classic
- ½ cup + 2 tbsp. coconut flour
- 1 ½ tsp. baking powder
- 2 zest of 2 lemons (reserve 1 tsp. for the glaze)
- 4 tsp. fresh lemon juice
- The Glaze:
- 2 tsp. freshly squeezed lemon juice
- 2 tbsp. Monkfruit Powder
- 1 tsp. lemon zest
- 1 splash heavy whipping cream

DIRECTIONS

1. Warm the oven to reach 325 degrees Fahrenheit. Prepare a bread pan using a layer of parchment baking paper.
2. Add the butter into a microwavable dish to melt. Let it cool.
3. Whisk the eggs, with the vanilla, heavy whipping cream, Monk fruit Classic, cream cheese, baking powder, and salt until combined.
4. Thoroughly mix in the coconut flour, melted butter, lemon zest, and juice to the mixture.
5. Scoop the batter into the prepared bread pan.
6. Bake it until the top of the bread is just beginning to brown and a toothpick inserted in the center comes out clean (55 min. to 1 hr.).
7. Prepare the glaze by combining the lemon juice with the Monkfruit Powder, lemon zest, and a splash of heavy whipping cream. Whisk until the glaze is creamy.
8. Empty the prepared glaze over the warm bread, spreading it out so that it covers the top and runs down the sides to serve.

NUTRITION

- Calories: 121
- Protein: g
- Carbs: 3g

- Fat: 10g
- Fiber: 1g

PREPARATION: 55 MIN

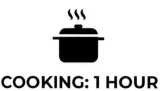
COOKING: 1 HOUR

SERVES: 16 REGULAR-SIZED CAKES

MOLTEN CHOCOLATE CAKE FROM CHILI'S

INGREDIENTS

- The Molten Lava Cakes:
- Caramel sauce
- Chocolate shell ice-cream topping
- Vanilla ice-cream
- ½ cup sour cream
- ½ cup oil
- 1 cup of milk
- 3 eggs
- 1 box fudge cake mix
- The Hot Fudge:
- 1 pinch salt
- 4 tbsp. of unsalted butter
- 12 oz. of semi-sweet chocolate chips
- 1 tsp. vanilla extract
- 14 oz. of sweetened condensed milk (see the keto recipe)
- The Magic Shell:
- ¼ cup of coconut oil
- 2 cups of chocolate chips

DIRECTIONS

1. Prepare The Lava Cakes:
2. Use a large mixing container to add the cake mix, oil, milk, sour cream, and eggs. Thoroughly mix.
3. Use a large non-stick cupcake pan and evenly distribute the batter ¾ of the way full.
4. Bake at 350 degrees Fahrenheit (25-30 min.)
5. Take out the cakes and allow them to cool down.
6. Take a knife, start cutting a hole at the center, and don't go till the bottom.
7. Pour the hot fudge into the hole that you made in the cake. Then take the piece of cake that you earlier removed while cutting the whole, slice off its bottom circle, and put it on the top of the hot fudge just like a lid.
8. Wrap the cake pan using a plastic layer to freeze for about 30 minutes, or for up to two days.
9. Reheat the cakes, after taking them out from the freezer, in the microwave for about 30 seconds until it's nice and warm.
10. Top the cakes with caramel, ice cream, and the magic shell.
11. The Hot Fudge:
12. Warm a saucepan using the medium-temperature setting before adding all the fudge fixings to melt.
13. Stir continuously and wait for them to boil.
14. Continue boiling and stirring for about two minutes.
15. Transfer the pan to a cool burner and stir. Let it cool.
16. The Magic Shell:
17. Use a microwave-proof bowl to add the coconut oil and chocolate. Heat it at thirty-second intervals in the microwave—while frequently stirring—until it is melted.
18. Serve it over the cold ice-cream and allow it to harden.

NUTRITION

- Calories: 723
- Carbs: 31g
- Protein: 9g
- Fat: 54g
- Fiber: 4g

CONCLUSION

Reaching Your Goal

The saying remains true—you will realize that what you put into your body will dictate how you feel. While on the Keto diet, you are building up energy stores for your body to utilize. That means that you should be feeling a necessary boost in your energy levels and the ability to pass each moment of each day without struggling. You can say goodbye to the sluggish feeling that often accompanies other diet plans. When you are on Keto, you should only be experiencing the benefits of additional energy and unlimited potential. Your diet isn't going to always feel like a diet. After some time, you will realize that you enjoy eating a Keto menu very much. Because your body will be switching the way it metabolizes, it will also change what it craves. Don't be surprised if you end up hungering fats and proteins as you progress on the Keto diet—this is what your body will eventually want.

Tracking Progress

Using a compare and contrast method is always great for monitoring progress. Remember how you felt before starting the Keto diet. If you haven't started already, you can use this time to document your current state of being. Make sure to record your mindset and the cravings that you have. When you have these figures to compare your progress to, you will use this as a motivating tool. Remember to allow yourself the feeling of pride as you make it through each day of being on the Keto diet. Commit yourself to the diet. That will present its own set of trials to face, but they will not be so complicated that you lose your way. Believe in your ability to see this through.

You Are What You Eat

Think about how you used to feel while eating your sugary and carb-loaded cravings. Your immediate response will likely suggest that you felt great but think about the bigger picture. Did you gain more energy from eating these things? Eating junk food only quietens your immediate cravings. When you think about it, this junk food indeed doesn't have a place in your life.

Choose to feel satisfied when you can know for sure that you are treating your body correctly. You should be able to handle the joy that comes from the fact that you are giving your body fuel that it can utilize. While eating your Keto-friendly food might not show you the same immediate rush that eating your favorite junk food does, it will benefit you much more in the long run. You will be able to notice its advantages long after you digest the food, which is essential. A simple change in perspective is what you need to realize that your happiness isn't directly tied to the cravings that you satisfy. Your satisfaction needs to stem from a deeper place.

Your Life Will Improve

There comes the point while being on the Keto diet that you make a shift from trying to succeeding. That will happen at various points for people, but when it happens to you, embrace it. Instead of concentrating on the fact that you are following a diet, you can begin to shift your focus to your receiving benefits. You need to ensure that you appreciate your life!

Your Body Will Change

One of the exciting benefits that you will begin enjoying is the way that your appearance will change. Your skin should have a healthy glow to it, appearing youthful. As the aging process takes place, feeling ashamed of your skin can become a prominent issue that impacts your self-esteem significantly. Aging is a process that no one is exempt from, but the Keto diet can help you do it more gracefully. When you notice that your skin is improving, you can commit to taking better care of it.

Your efforts should not only inspire those around you, but they should also serve as a way to motivate yourself. Acknowledge your progress and recognize the challenges that you had to face while arriving there. You will wonder what you even used to eat before. That is why Keto tends to be a permanent solution. Even those who agree to try it for a few months end up sticking with it for much longer. Just keep it up unless it no longer feels right. If you are getting all of your benefits plus the satisfaction of being full of eating clean foods, you will likely continue feeling great while on Keto.

Made in the USA
Columbia, SC
29 July 2021